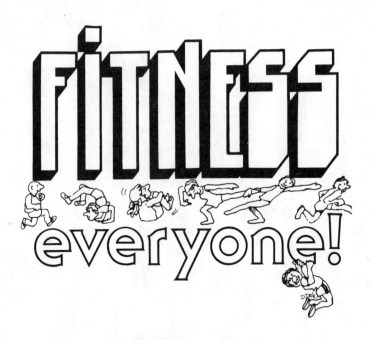

FITNESS everyone!

Roberta Stokes
D. Delzingro Farls

Miami-Dade Community College
Miami, Florida

Hunter Textbooks Inc.

©1983 by Hunter Textbooks Inc.

ISBN 0-89459-200-9

Printed in the United States of America

Inquiries should be addressed to
the publisher:

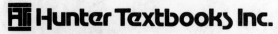

Hunter Textbooks Inc.

823 Reynolda Road
Winston-Salem, North Carolina 27104

PREFACE

Interest in health and personal fitness is rapidly increasing among all Americans. People are recognizing the importance of achieving optimal levels of fitness rather than being satisfied with just being average. In attempting to reshape and change their bodies, Americans increasingly are setting personal goals and accepting responsibility for making changes in their lifestyle.

The authors offer this text as accurate, current information to assist every person to achieve optimal fitness. In addition to providing guidelines for nutrition and exercise, examples of practical exercise programs, answers to commonly asked questions, and hints for stress reduction and relaxation, this book is unique in another facet. It includes the usual areas for fitness — flexibility, strength, and cardiovascular — but it also emphasizes the role aerobic dance plays in achieving fitness.

Our major objective is to challenge each reader to reach high — to seek the highest possible level of health and fitness.

The question: "Is your current lifestyle worth dying for?" Why not make the commitment to change today? The choice is yours!

ACKNOWLEDGMENTS

The authors gratefully acknowledge the many suggestions and ideas contributed by their colleagues.

Special credit is due the Figure Improvement instructors at Miami-Dade
Community College South for their assistance with various portions of this text.
Grateful acknowledgment is also given to Barbara Bullock, Carol Brown, and
Christi Hurwitz, who typed the manuscript.

Contents

Chapter 1

SEEING THE WHOLE PICTURE
■
Optimal Fitness

The word fitness means different things to different people. There are various levels of fitness and various components of fitness. Optimal fitness refers to the attainment of one's highest possible level of overall health. Unfortunately, the average person does not live at an optimal level of health or fitness. Most seem satisfied to reach minimal standards rather than attaining the highest attainable level of health — optimal fitness. Our error in the past has been in believing that reaching a "normal" or average level implied we were in good health. We now know that such standards are misleading because our population has a high incidence of obesity, hypertension, smoking; a poor level of physical fitness; and a diet high in calories, fat, and cholesterol. Therefore, only by seeking optimal standards can we be assured of the highest level of health.

The key to attaining an optimal level of health and fitness is a change in lifestyle. There is little doubt that our modern lifestyle contributes to being unfit but this can be changed. We can make different choices in regard to exercise, smoking, diet, and control of stress, but we need to initiate these changes as early as possible. The evidence is clear that we can affect our chances of living at almost any time in our lives, but the earlier we start the greater the effect will be.

How can we achieve optimal fitness? First, we must analyze our behavior and lifestyle to determine what changes need to be made. Second, we need to evaluate our current fitness level to identify strengths and weaknesses; and third, we must establish goals for improvement, then plan and follow an individualized training program.

Lifestyle Changes

Three important areas in lifestyle should be examined for possible change: activity, diet, and stress.

The problem in today's sedentary society is that our daily tasks of living no longer require rigorous physical activity. In addition, most of us usually look for every possible way of avoiding exercise — we ride rather than walk, use

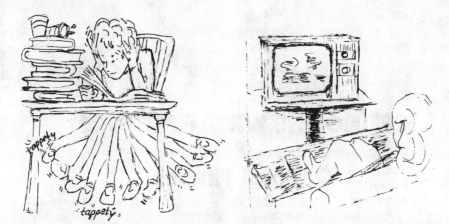

elevators instead of stairs, sit and watch television rather than be active, and use every labor-saving device possible. We simply must turn this around so that activity becomes a regular part of our lives.

Exercise can be planned to fit into any busy schedule and become a daily habit. Our daily nutritional habits also need review. We can bring our intake of nutrients in line with those recommended for optimal nutrition. We can eliminate or decrease excessive calories, fat, cholesterol, sugar, and salt from our diet. Dietary habits are not easy to change but the choice is ours.

Another area of lifestyle which must be examined is the control of stress. The increased pressures brought about by the complexities of modern civilization are taking a tremendous toll on most Americans.

The stress of our lifestyles contributes to and is associated with numerous psychological and even physical disorders. We must become more aware of stress factors and learn how to cope with them. There are effective techniques that can be employed if the problem is first identified.

If your motivation is strong enough, you can make the changes in your lifestyle that will help you achieve optimal fitness.

Fitness Evaluation

Numerous tests have indicated the general lack of minimal levels of physical fitness among American children and adults. As a nation we have not recognized the necessity of regular exercise for our personal health and well-being. Regardless of age, we now must take the time to learn how to evaluate individual strengths and weaknesses. We need to know which specific areas of our personal fitness need improvement and then we can set realistic goals for change. There are four major components of physical fitness relating directly to a person's health: cardiovascular endurance, flexibility, muscular strength and endurance, and body composition.

Cardiovascular endurance is the most important element of physical fitness. It is a measure of the ability of your heart, lungs, and blood vessels to function effectively. A high level of cardiovascular endurance is essential, not only to achieving fitness but to the performance of our everyday activities.

Flexibility is the capacity of a joint to move through its normal range of motion. Lack of flexibility may result in postural problems, muscle injury and soreness, limitation of movement, inability to perform daily tasks, and restricted performance of many sport skills. Studies show that the most frequent cause of loss of flexibility is lack of continued exercise.

Muscular strength and endurance are closely related components of fitness. Strength refers to the ability of a muscle to exert force against resistance. Muscular endurance is the ability of a muscle to exert force continuously over a period of time. Therefore if a muscle grows stronger its ability to continue to contract without fatigue will be greater. Increased muscular endurance will enable you to perform simple household tasks more effectively and improve your sports performance. In addition, muscles that are stronger will be less susceptible to injury from strains and sprains. Since fitness is not a static condition but a constantly changing one, we must periodically reassess our status. That is one of the challenges that achieving fitness presents — **we must make a lifelong commitment to it.**

Body composition refers to the percentage of body weight that is fat in relation to that which is lean muscle mass. Excessive accumulation of body fat (obesity) is closely related to many physical and emotional problems. If you are to reach your state of optimal fitness, body weight and percentage of fat must be kept within an acceptable range.

The Training Program

Perhaps the key to obtaining optimal fitness is the establishment of specific goals and the commitment to an individualized training program. You must develop a positive plan for changing your lifestyle in all areas and actually participate in a regular exercise program. Since exercise is an individual thing, a variety of training programs can be followed. The important thing is to find the one that is "right" for you — the one that meets your needs and interests, the one you can stay with throughout your life. Of course, exercise alone cannot do it all, but it certainly is a proven method for attaining a high level of fitness.

There is no doubt that a commitment to change your lifestyle will require time, effort, and sacrifice. Along the way you may experience discouragement, doubt, and failure. However, if you can keep in mind the benefits of reaching a goal of optimal fitness it may help you to maintain your determination. Some of the specific outcomes of achieving optimal fitness and participating in a regular program of physical activity include:

1. You will have more energy.

2. It helps you cope with stress.

3. It increases your resistance to fatigue.

4.   It improves your self-image.

5.   It helps your relax and feel less tense.

6.   Your muscles will remain firm.

7.   Your heart and lungs will function more efficiently.

8.   There is a decrease in body fat.

9.   The aging process is delayed.

10.   You will have an increased physical work capacity.

Chapter 2 will start you toward your goal by suggesting evaluation methods to assess your current level of fitness.

REFERENCES

1.   Allsen, P.; Harrison, J.; and Vance, B.. *Fitness for Life*. Wm. C. Brown Co. Dubuque, Iowa, 1980.

2.   Falls, H.; Baylor, A; and Dishman, R. *Essentials of Fitness*. Saunders College, Philadelphia, 1980.

3.   Garrison, L.; Leslie, P; and Blackmore, D. *Fitness and Figure Control*. Mayfield Publishing Co., Palo Alto, California, 1981.

4.   Getchell, Bud. *Being Fit — A Personal Guide*. John Wiley & Sons, New York, 1982.

5.   Getchell, Bud. *Physical Fitness: A Way of Life*. John Wiley & Sons, New York, 1976.

6.   Golding, L.; Myers, C.; and Sinning, W. (eds). *The Y's Way to Physical Fitness*. National Board of YMCA, Chicago, 1982.

7.   Hockey, Robert V. *Physical Fitness — The Pathway to Healthful Living*. C. V. Mosby Co., St. Louis, 1981.

8.   Miller, David and Allen, T. Earl. *Fitness: A Lifetime Commitment*. Burgess Publishing Co., Minneapolis, 1982.

9.   U.S. Dept. of Health & Human Services. *Exercise and Your Heart*. U.S. Government Printing Office, 1981.

Chapter 2

UNDERSTANDING THE PROBLEM
■
Assessment of Current Fitness

How physically fit are you? Are you in good overall health? Have you had a physical examination recently? How active have you been? Can you perform daily activities without tiring easily? Do you have an acceptable level of body fat? These are important questions which need to be examined before beginning an exercise program.

Assessment of your current fitness level should begin with a review of your family and personal health history. Laboratory Report 2 contains a sample health questionnaire. Its purpose is to detect disorders that might prevent or restrict your participation in a regular exercise program, and to evaluate your degree of heart attack risk. It is extremely important that all questions be answered as accurately as possible so that an effective and safe individual program might be developed. If there are any doubts about the advisability of your participation in an exercise program you should first consult with a medical doctor.

The next step is to determine your current physical condition so that personal improvement goals, and an appropriate training program can be designed. This can be accomplished by participating in a series of physical fitness tests. Since physical fitness is composed of several factors, a variety of tests are needed to evaluate them. You may score well on some tests and poorly on others. Hopefully the test results will motivate you to seek improvement and establish a regular exercise program. By repeating the tests periodically, you can evaluate your progress and determine the effectiveness of your training program.

After completing the tests and activities which are described, you will be able to establish your physical fitness profile by utilizing the charts in this chapter. These charts will help you compare your results to others of your age and sex who have previously completed the tests. However, the establishment of precise test norms and standards is difficult and therefore norms should only be used as a guide to your particular strengths and weaknesses — not as a means of comparing yourself to others. Actually you should concentrate on improving your scores and measure your own individual improvement. You should establish a goal of "optimal" physical fitness for *you*. The optimal level refers to the achievement of your maximum potential. Each of us is unique and will improve at a different rate, so do not become discouraged if others seem to develop more quickly than you. Just strive to do the best you can and continue to progress toward your goal.

EVALUATING CARDIOVASCULAR ENDURANCE

Cardiovascular endurance is a measure of the ability of the heart to pump blood, of the lungs to process volumes of air, and of the muscles to utilize oxygen. Tests designed to measure cardiovascular endurance involve vigorous physical activity that make high demands on the heart and lungs. One's level of cardiovascular endurance is generally considered the most important single measure of the overall level of fitness because it reflects the condition of the heart, blood vessels, and lungs as well as the general condition of the muscles.

Walking Test

For those individuals who are considerably overweight, who have been inactive for some time, or are over 35 years of age, it is recommended that a walking test be attempted before more strenuous cardiovascular tests. This test simply consists of pre-measuring a distance of one mile and then timing yourself on how long it takes you to walk the distance. If you cannot complete the one mile or if it takes you longer than 15 minutes, it indicates you have a very low level of fitness. Depending on your test results and how you feel when you finished, you may find it necessary to begin a walking program before taking a running test.

Run-Walk Tests

12 Minute Run-Walk Test. One simple test for measuring cardiovascular endurance is the 12 minute run-walk test. This test has been found to give a reliable estimate of one's maximal oxygen consumption and can be used in place of more extensive tests such as the treadmill or bicycle ergometer test. The test involves measuring the distance covered by running, or running and walking, for 12 minutes. The purpose is to cover as much distance as possible; however, the test should not be continued if extreme fatigue, dizziness, shortness of breath, or nausea are experienced. Ratings of your cardiovascular endurance based on the 12 minute run-walk are on the opposite page.

1.5 Mile Run-Walk Test. An alternate test for determining cardiovascular endurance is the 1.5 mile run-walk test. The time it takes the individual to run-walk a distance of 1.5 miles is recorded to the nearest hundredth of a second. One should observe the same precautions as with the 12 minute run-walk test, but attempt to cover the distance in the shortest possible time.

Ratings of cardiovascular endurance based on the 1.5 mile run-walk are given on the opposite page.

12-MINUTE RUN-WALK RATINGS

RATING	FEMALES (BY AGE)					
	13-19	20-29	30-39	40-49	50-59	60+
Superior	>1.52	>1.46	>1.40	>1.35	>1.31	>1.19
Excellent	1.44-1.51	1.35-1.45	1.30-1.39	1.25-1.34	1.19-1.30	1.10-1.18
Good	1.30-1.43	1.23-1.34	1.19-1.29	1.12-1.24	1.06-1.18	.99-1.09
Fair	1.19-1.29	1.12-1.22	1.06-1.18	.99-1.11	.94-1.05	.87-.98
Poor	1.00-1.18	.96-1.11	.95-1.05	.88-.98	.84-.93	.78-.86
Very Poor	<1.00	<.96	<.95	<.88	<.84	<.78

RATING	MALES (BY AGE)					
	13-19	20-29	30-39	40-49	50-59	60+
Superior	>1.87	>1.77	>1.70	>1.66	>1.59	>1.56
Excellent	1.73-1.86	1.65-1.76	1.57-1.69	1.54-1.65	1.45-1.58	1.33-1.55
Good	1.57-1.72	1.50-1.64	1.46-1.56	1.40-1.53	1.31-1.44	1.21-1.32
Fair	1.38-1.56	1.32-1.49	1.31-1.45	1.25-1.39	1.17-1.30	1.03-1.20
Poor	1.30-1.37	1.22-1.31	1.18-1.30	1.14-1.24	1.03-1.16	.87-1.02
Very Poor	<1.30	<1.22	<1.18	<1.14	<1.03	<.87

1.5 MILE RUN RATINGS

FITNESS CATEGORY	FEMALES (BY AGE)					
	13-19	20-29	30-39	40-49	50-59	60+
Superior	>11:50	>12:30	>13:00	>13:45	>14:30	>16:30
Excellent	11:50-12:29	12:30-13:30	13:00-14:30	13:45-15:55	14:30-16:30	16:30-17:30
Good	12:30-14:30	13:31-15:54	14:31-16:30	15:56-17:30	16:31-19:00	17:31-19:30
Fair	14:31-16:54	15:55-18:30	16:31-19:00	17:31-19:30	19:01-20:00	19:31-20:30
Poor	16:55-18:30	18:31-19:00	19:01-19:30	19:31-20:00	20:01-20:30	20:31-21:00
Very Poor	<18:31	<19:01	<19:31	<20:01	<20:31	<21:01

FITNESS CATEGORY	MALES (BY AGE)					
	13-19	20-29	30-39	40-49	50-59	60+
Superior	<8:37	<9:45	<10:00	<10:30	<11:00	<11:15
Excellent	8:37-9:40	9:45-10:45	10:00-11:00	10:30-11:30	11:00-12:30	11:15-13:59
Good	9:41-10:48	10:46-12:00	11:01-12:30	11:31-13:00	12:31-14:30	14:00-16:15
Fair	10:49-12:10	12:01-14:00	12:31-14:45	13:01-15:35	14:31-17:00	16:16-19:00
Poor	12:11-15:30	14:01-16:00	14:46-16:30	15:36-17:30	17:01-19:00	19:01-20:00
Very Poor	>15:31	>16:10	>16:31	>17:31	>19:01	>20:01

> = more than   < = less than

Resting Heart Rate

Another measure of cardiovascular efficiency is the resting heart rate. The best way to measure the resting heart rate is to take the pulse upon waking in the morning, and while still in bed. The resting pulse may also be measured by selecting a time when you have not done any physical activity for at least 30 minutes, have not eaten for several hours, and feel relaxed. A lower resting heart rate is desired since it is an indication that the heart is working more efficiently in meeting the body's demand for blood. It also means a greater stroke volume, which indicates that more blood is pumped with each beat allowing the heart more time for rests between beats. Studies show that people who develop high levels of cardiovascular endurance often have resting heart rates below 50 beats per minute. The American Heart Association identifies the normal range for resting heart rates as being between 50-100 beats per minute. The resting heart rate will decrease gradually in response to a program of regular endurance activities. By keeping a record of your resting pulse rate, you can chart the progress you are making in your training program.

Counting Your Pulse

The pulse can be counted most accurately by applying light pressure to the radial artery on the inside of your wrist. Place the tips of the first two fingers on the wrist just below the base of the thumb and press lightly. When you feel the pulse, count the number of beats for the appropriate time period using a stop watch or a watch with a second hand. An alternate spot for finding the pulse is the carotid artery which is found by placing two fingers lightly under the jawbone slightly to the back of the Adam's apple.

Heart Rate Recovery Test (Sit-Stand)

The purpose of this test is to measure cardiovascular efficiency through a simple test of sitting and standing for three minutes while keeping a record of heart rate at various stages. Determination of one's recovery heart rate is an indication of the condition of the heart, lungs, blood vessels, and working muscles. The person with a higher level of cardiovascular fitness will have a smaller increase in heart rate and, following the test, the heart rate will return to normal faster than a person who has a lower level of cardiovascular fitness.

In this test the subject sits and stands 24 times a minute for 3 minutes with the arms folded in front of the body. The heart rate is recorded at rest, immediately after exercise and 30 seconds, one minute, and two minutes later. The results enable a person to determine the general fitness zone which they are in: danger zone, safety zone, or fitness zone. The recording form for the test and rating chart are found on the next page. This test is not as strenuous as the run-walk tests and may serve as an effective screening test for cardiovascular efficiency.

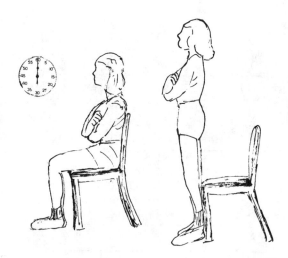

HEART RATE RECOVERY TEST: SIT/STAND
Procedure

1. Record resting heart rate by taking pulse for 15 seconds. Record rate on the score card.

2. Starting from a sitting position with arms folded, stand up and sit down twice every 5 seconds (24 times each minute) for 3 minutes.

3. At the end of 3 minutes sit down quickly and find your pulse. Count the heart rate for 15 seconds and record it as the immediate Post-test Heart Rate index.

4. The 30 Second Recovery Heart Rate is recorded after taking the pulse once again for 15 seconds (from 30-45 seconds after the exercise).

5. The One-Minute Recovery Heart Rate is recorded in the same manner as the 30 Second Recovery Heart Rate.

6. The Two-Minute Recovery Heart Rate is recorded by taking the pulse for 15 seconds after two full minutes of rest.

7. Multiply all pulse scores by 4 as indicated on the score sheet.

8. Circle the heart rate scores on the chart and find the codes directly above the circled heart rates. Write the codes in the space provided to the right of the chart.

9. Add the codes for all 5 heart rates and circle the total code score which indicates your fitness zone.

HEART RATE RECOVERY (SIT/STAND TEST) *

CODING YOUR CARDIOVASCULAR HEALTH CODES

	20	19	18	17	16	15	14	13	12	11	10	9	8	7	6	5	4	3	2	1	Code Score
×4 Score — Starting Heart Rate	44	48	52	56	60	62	64	66	68	70	72	74	76	78	80	84	88	92	96	100	___
×4 Score — Post-test Heart Rate	80	84	88	92	96	100	104	108	112	116	120	124	128	132	136	140	144	148	152	156	___
×4 Score — 30-Second Recovery Heart Rate	64	68	72	76	80	84	88	92	96	100	104	108	112	116	120	124	128	132	136	140	___
×4 Score — 1-Minute Recovery Heart Rate	56	60	64	68	72	76	80	84	88	92	96	100	104	108	112	116	120	124	128	132	___
×4 Score — 2-Minute Recovery Heart Rate	56	60	64	68	72	76	80	84	88	92	96	100	104	108	112	116	120	124	128	132	___

Results

0-35 = Danger Zone
36-70 = Safety Zone
71-100 = Fitness Zone

Total Code Scores ═══

* Pipes, T.V. Vodak, P.A. *The Pipes Fitness Test and Prescription*, New York: St. Martin's Press, 1978.

EVALUATING BODY COMPOSITION

Information about your body proportions, distribution of fatty deposits, and total body fat percentage is needed to help determine your ideal body weight. As will be discussed in Chapter 6, standard height-weight tables can be very misleading since they do not distinguish between weight that is fat and weight that is lean muscle mass. Studies indicate a direct relationship between excess amounts of fat and low levels of physical fitness and a higher risk of cardiovascular disease. A complete analysis of your body composition should therefore include height and body weight, selected girth measurements, and body fat percentage.

Girth Measurement

By measuring the girth of certain areas of the body, you can determine your relative trimness and the relationship of your body proportions to those desired. This is usually an area of high interest since our body proportions determine how we look to others and ourselves.

In order to obtain accurate measurements, you should have another person take your measurements with a standard cloth tape measure and record them. While being measured you should stand relaxed and breathe normally with the weight evenly distributed on both feet. The tape measure should be carefully placed around each area so that it remains parallel to the ground and is not applied too tightly. The tissue underneath should not be indented or compressed.

The chart on the next page indicates the exact sites for your measurements and the recommended girth proportions for men and women. Keep in mind that the recommended proportions can only be used as general guidelines for achieving a trim, well-proportioned body. (3)

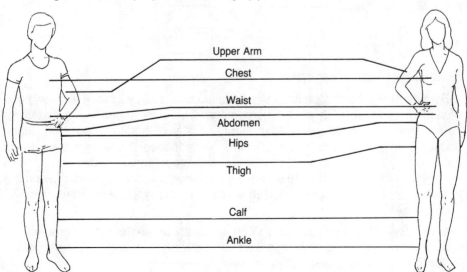

Upper Arm

Chest

Waist

Abdomen

Hips

Thigh

Calf

Ankle

GIRTH MEASUREMENT (3)

Site	Recommended Proportion	
	Men	Women
CHEST (Bust) - at the nipple level	Same as hips	Same as hips
WAIST - Below the rib cage above the top of the hip bone (at the minimal· abdominal area)	5-7 inches less than chest or hips	10 inches less than bust or hips
ABDOMEN - Just below the navel, the largest girth between the waist and hips	1 1/2 inches smaller than the chest	2 1/2 inches smaller than bust
HIPS - The maximum girth of the buttocks below the hip bone in front	Same as chest	Same as bust
THIGH - An inch or two below the crotch at the largest girth	8-10 inches less than waist	6 inches less than waist
CALF - the largest girth	7-8 inches less than thighs	6-7 inches less than thighs
ANKLE - The smallest girth just above the ankle bone	6-7 inches less than calves	5-6 inches less than calves
UPPER ARM - The largest girth when the arm is held relaxed with forearm parallel to the floor and palm up	Twice the size of the wrist	Twice the size of the wrist
WRIST - The smallest girth when the arm is held with forearm parallel to the floor and palm up	—	—

Body Fat Measurements

By measuring the thickness of skinfolds at various body sites, it is possible to obtain an estimate of body fat percentage. This assessment is important in helping you determine the relative leanness of your body composition. Since accurate measurement by individuals experienced in using calipers is necessary, you may not be able to obtain such a percentage. However, you can be certain that if you pinch one of the designated areas (see Appendix A) and the measurement is more than one inch across the fold, you have a high body fat percentage.

Laboratory 5 provides specific information about skinfold measurement as well as norm tables to determine an estimate of your body fat percentage. Percentages are classified in the following chart.

BODY FAT CLASSIFICATION

Classification	Percent Fat	
	Male	Female
Very Lean	10%	13%
Lean	11-15%	14-18%
Average	16-19%	19-22%
Fat	20-24%	23-27%
Very Fat	25% over	28% over

Determining Your Target Weight

No doubt one of your primary concerns is how much you should weigh. Chapter 6 points out the problem with using standard height-weight tables that indicate desirable weight based on averages taken from general insurance population statistics. These tables do not consider the percentage of body fat and therefore can be very misleading. A commonly used height-weight table developed by the U.S. Dept of Agriculture provides a more realistic guide for determining desirable weight. These charts are shown on page 15.

Once you have determined your percentage of body fat a more accurate calculation of "ideal" or target weight can be made. Use the example below to establish your target weight.

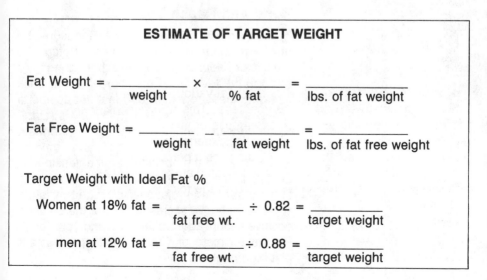

ESTIMATE OF TARGET WEIGHT

Fat Weight = _____ × _____ = _____
              weight   % fat   lbs. of fat weight

Fat Free Weight = _____ − _____ = _____
                   weight   fat weight lbs. of fat free weight

Target Weight with Ideal Fat %

Women at 18% fat = _____ ÷ 0.82 = _____
                    fat free wt.   target weight

men at 12% fat = _____ ÷ 0.88 = _____
                  fat free wt.   target weight

EXAMPLE OF TARGET WEIGHT

Fat Weight = $\dfrac{140}{\text{weight}}$ × $\dfrac{.25}{\text{\% fat}}$ = $\dfrac{35}{\text{lbs. of fat weight}}$

Fat Free Weight = $\dfrac{140}{\text{weight}}$ − $\dfrac{35}{\text{fat weight}}$ = $\dfrac{105}{\text{lbs. of fat free weight}}$

Target Weight with Ideal Fat %

Women at 18% fat = $\dfrac{105}{\text{fat free wt.}}$ ÷ 0.82 = $\dfrac{128\,\text{lbs.}}{\text{target weight}}$

men at 12% fat = $\dfrac{105}{\text{fat free wt.}}$ ÷ 0.88 = $\dfrac{119\,\text{lbs.}}{\text{target weight}}$

EVALUATING FLEXIBILITY

Flexibility is the ability of an individual to move the various body joints through a maximum range of motion. It is an important aspect of physical fitness, and the lack of flexibility can lead to numerous physical disorders and problems. Basically, the loss of flexibility is due to the lack of muscle use. Loss of flexibility can limit one's movements and ability to perform daily tasks as well as recreational activities. No single test can measure flexibility since it is specific to each joint and muscle group. However, the following tests do provide an indication of flexibility for various parts of the body.

Bend and Reach Test

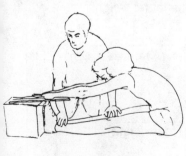

The purpose of this test is to measure the ability to bend your trunk and stretch the muscles of your back and your hamstrings. To perform the test, sit on the floor with your back straight, knees together, and feet flat against a box. As a partner holds your knees straight, reach forward with the arms fully extended, palms down, fingers straight and thumbs touching. Hold the position at full extension for at least three seconds. The distance the fingertips reach in relationship to the box is the score — negative scores in front of the box and positive scores beyond the box (and your toes). Ratings for your bend and reach test scores are given on page 16.

DESIRABLE WEIGHTS FOR WOMEN
Weights listed without clothing according to height without shoes. (From U.S. Department of Agriculture, *Food and Your Weight,* Washington, D.C.: U.S. Government Printing Office, 1973)

Height (feet, inches)	Below Average	Weight (lbs.) Average	Above Average
5 - 0	100	109	118
5 - 1	104	112	121
5 - 2	107	115	125
5 - 3	110	118	128
5 - 4	113	122	132
5 - 5	116	125	135
5 - 6	120	129	139
5 - 7	123	132	142
5 - 8	126	136	146
5 - 9	130	140	151
5 - 10	133	144	156
5 - 11	137	148	161
6 - 0	141	152	166

DESIRABLE WEIGHTS FOR MEN
Weights listed without clothing according to height without shoes. (From U.S. Department of Agriculture, *Food and Your Weight,* Washington, D.C.: U.S. Government Printing Office, 1973)

Height (feet, inches)	Below Average	Weight (lbs.) Average	Above Average
5 - 0	100	109	118
5 - 1	104	112	121
5 - 2	107	115	125
5 - 3	110	118	128
5 - 4	113	122	132
5 - 5	116	125	135
5 - 6	120	129	139
5 - 7	123	132	142
5 - 8	126	136	146
5 - 9	130	140	151
5 - 10	133	144	156
5 - 11	137	148	161
6 - 0	141	152	166

Bend and Reach Test

FITNESS CATEGORY	MALES	FEMALES
Superior	> 8	> 8
Excellent	6-7	6-7
Good	4-5	4-5
Average	2-3	2-3
Fair	0-1	0-1
Poor	< 0	< 0

Trunk Extension Test

FITNESS CATEGORY	MALES	FEMALES
Superior	> 24	> 22
Excellent	22-23	20-21
Good	20-21	17-19
Average	18-19	15-16
Fair	16-17	13-14
Poor	< 16	< 13

Shoulder Lift

FITNESS CATEGORY	MALES	FEMALES
Superior	> 28	> 27
Excellent	26-27	25-26
Good	24-25	22-24
Average	22-23	19-21
Fair	20-21	17-18
Poor	< 19	< 17

> = more than   < = less than

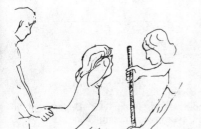

Trunk Extension Test

The purpose of this test is to measure the flexibility of the trunk by arching the back from the prone position. To perform the test, lie prone on the floor with a partner holding the buttocks and legs down. Interlock your fingers behind your neck with your elbows outward and raise your chest and head off the floor as high as possible. The distance from the floor to the bottom of your chin is the score. Ratings for the trunk extension test score are given above.

Shoulder Lift Test

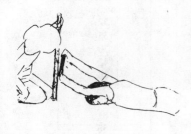

The purpose of this test is to measure the range of motion of the shoulder joint. To perform the test, lie prone on the floor with the chin and forehead touching the floor and the arms extended forward directly in front of the shoulders with a stick or ruler held in both hands. With a partner holding the buttocks and legs down and keeping the chin on the floor, measure the distance from the bottom of the stick or ruler to the floor. Ratings for the shoulder lift test score are given above.

EVALUATING MUSCULAR ENDURANCE

Muscular endurance is a measure of the ability of a specific muscle group to exert force repeatedly or the ability to maintain a given muscle contraction for a period of time. Minimal muscular strength (the ability to apply force) and muscular endurance are needed for everyday tasks, for recreational activities, and to prevent posture problems which are related to muscular weakness, such as lower back pain. Performance on such tests can be affected by one's height, weight, and fatness, but they can provide reasonable estimates of your body strength and muscular endurance.

Bent Knee Sit-Up Test

The purpose of this test is to measure the muscular endurance of the abdominal muscles. To perform the test, lie on your back face up with fingers interlocked behind your head. Both feet are placed flat on the floor, with knees flexed at approximately a 90° angle. An assistant holds your feet firmly in place as you sit up to a position with the back perpendicular to the floor and then return to the floor so that your hands contact the floor. The number of sit-ups completed in one minute is the score. Ratings for your sit-up test score follow.

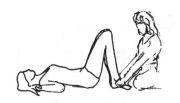

FITNESS CATEGORY	BENT KNEE SIT-UP RATINGS MALES (by age)				
	20-29	30-39	40-49	50-59	60-69
Excellent	48 above	40 above	35 above	30 above	25 above
Good	43-47	35-39	30-34	25-29	20-24
Average	37-42	29-34	24-29	19-24	14-19
Fair	33-36	25-28	20-23	15-18	10-13
Poor	0-32	0-24	0-19	0-14	0-9

FITNESS CATEGORY	BENT KNEE SIT-UP RATINGS FEMALES (by age)				
	20-29	30-39	40-49	50-59	60-69
Excellent	44 above	36 above	31 above	26 above	21 above
Good	39-43	31-35	26-30	21-25	16-20
Average	33-38	25-30	19-25	15-20	10-15
Fair	29-32	21-24	16-18	11-14	6-9
Poor	0-28	0-20	0-15	0-10	0-5

Push-up

The purpose of this test is to measure the muscular endurance of the muscles in the arm and shoulder area. To perform the test assume a front-leaning position on the floor with the hands directly under your shoulders, legs straight and toes tucked to support the body. The body is lowered by bending the elbows until the chin or chest touches the floor and then immediately returned to the starting position. Throughout the test the body is kept in a straight line from head to toe. The number of correct push-ups one can perform continuously is the score. Ratings for your push-up test score follow.

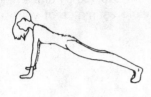

PUSH-UP RATINGS

FITNESS CATEGORY	MALES (by age)					FEMALES	
	20-29	30-39	40-49	50-59	60-69	Rating	Push-Up
Excellent	55 above	45 above	40 above	35 above	30 above	Excellent	27 up
Good	45-54	35-44	30-39	25-34	20-29	Good	19-26
Average	35-44	25-34	20-29	15-24	10-19	Average	12-18
Fair	20-34	15-24	12-19	8-14	5-9	Fair	5-11
Poor	0-19	0-14	0-11	0-7	0-4	Poor	0-4

Static Push-up

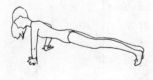

The purpose of this test is to serve as an alternate test for the regular push-up test. It is particularly appropriate for women who lack arm strength. To perform the test assume a front-leaning position on the floor with the hands directly under your shoulders, legs straight, and toes tucked to support the body. The body is lowered until the elbows are flexed to 90° or less and held in this position as long as possible. The test is complete when any part of the body touches the floor or the body is not held parallel to the floor. The score is determined by clocking the time in total seconds that the correct position is held. Ratings for your static push-up test score follow. (3)

STATIC PUSH-UP RATINGS

MALES		FEMALES	
Rating	Total Time Held	Rating	Total Time Held
Excellent	111 sec. - above	Excellent	35 sec. - above
Good	102-110 sec.	Good	30-34 sec.
Average	97-101 sec.	Average	26-29 sec.
Fair	88-96 sec.	Fair	20-25 sec.
Poor	0-87 sec.	Poor	0-19 sec.

Analyzing the Results

Once you have completed the testing, the results can be used to prepare an individual fitness profile (see Lab 3). This profile will indicate your specific strengths and weaknesses and provide the direction needed to develop an individualized physical improvement program. The next chapter will provide help in designing a program that is safe and effective.

REFERENCES

1. Cooper, Kenneth. *The Aerobics Way.* Bantam Books, New York, 1977.

2. Elrick, H; Crakes, J.; and Clarke, S. *Living Longer and Better.* World Publications, Mountain View, California, 1978.

3. Getchell, Bud. *Being Fit — A Personal Guide.* John Wiley & Sons, New York, 1982.

4. Getchell, Bud. *Physical Fitness: A Way of Life.* John Wiley & Sons, New York, 1976.

5. Golding, L.; Myers, C.; and Sinning, W. (eds.) *The Y's Way to Physical Fitness.* National Board of YMCA, Chicago, 1982.

6. Hockey, Robert V. *Physical Fitness — The Pathway to Healthful Living.* C.V. Mosby Co., St. Louis, 1981.

7. Lindsey, R.; Jones, B.; and Whitley, A. *Body Mechanics.* Wm. C. Brown Co., Dubuque, Iowa, 1979.

8. Miller, David K. and Allen, T. Earl. *Fitness: A Lifetime Commitment.* Burgess Publishing Co., Minneapolis, 1982.

Chapter 3

GETTING STARTED
■
Training Programs

Now that you have gained an understanding of your current fitness level, you are ready to develop a program that will help you reach your highest level of fitness. Your optimal level relates to your particular interests, needs, and abilities. Each of us is different but, regardless of our previous experience, disease or disability, every person can improve his or her health and strive for optimal fitness. It is not important to compare yourself to others — seek to achieve the highest level possible for you.

Success in reaching this level will depend to a large extent on the training program you utilize. Unfortunately many people with good intentions become frustrated and fall short of their goal because of basic fallacies in their training program. By observing certain principles and guidelines you can safely engage in a program that will provide maximum results.

Principles of Training

FREQUENCY

OCTOBER

						1
2	3	4	5	6	7	8
9	**10**	11	12	13	14	15
16	17	18	19	20	21	22
23	24	25	26	27	28	29
30	31					

At least 3 times per week

Exercise must be performed on a regular basis if it is to be effective. Hopefully, exercise will become a part of your daily lifestyle; however, benefits can be achieved with at least **three work-outs per week.** The work-outs should be spaced throughout the week rather than on consecutive days. A frequency of four or five times per week will produce a greater caloric expenditure.

INTENSITY

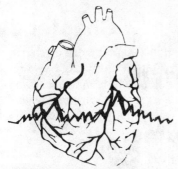

Achieve your target heart rate

Exercise must be strenuous enough to require more effort than usual. As the body adapts to this work load, an increased demand can be placed upon it.

The intensity needed to produce improvement will vary depending upon the current physical condition of the individual. In a poorly conditioned person, walking may be strenuous enough to produce a training effect.

One can accurately determine the intensity of a cardiovascular work-out by measuring the exercise heart rate. In addition, one should listen to his/her body. Your body will tell you when you are exercising too long and too hard.

DURATION (TIME)

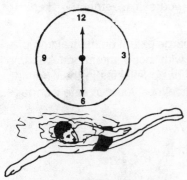

A 30 minute work-out is recommended (minimum)

In order to be effective exercise must be maintained for a significant length of time. A 30 minute work-out allows for sufficient warm-up and cool-down with at least 15 minutes at the target heart rate level. If you only exercise three times a week, the total duration should be extended by 10-15 minutes to increase the caloric expenditure for the week.

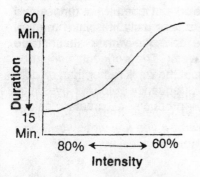

Exercise duration and intensity are directly related. Therefore, an activity performed at a higher intensity can be done for a shorter duration (with 15 minutes a day at a higher intensity as the minimum duration). The duration must be increased for those activities done at a lower intensity, i.e., walking.

Determining Target Heart Rate

In order to reach the necessary intensity it has been noted that you exercise in your target heart rate zone. For most young adults, a target heart rate between 150-170 beats per minute will achieve this intensity. Older adults may only need to achieve a rate between 130-140 beats per minute to reach their target heart rate zone. To determine your specific target heart rate you should follow these easy steps.

220	(MHR The maximum heart rate you can achieve during exercise)
– _____	(Your age - the MHR decreases as one gets older)
= _____	(Your MHR)
– _____	(Your resting heart rate)
= _____	(Heart rate reserve)
× .75 _____	(75% – work-out intensity - between 60 & 80% is recommended)
= _____	
+ _____	(Your resting heart rate)
= _____	Target Heart Rate at the 75% level

By determining your target heart rate zone, you can be certain you are achieving a high enough intensity to benefit from the work-out and yet not be pushing yourself too hard. Exercising within your target zone should not make you feel greatly uncomfortable. If you feel overly tired, try working at a lower rate until you are ready to progress to a higher zone.

Since it is difficult to count your pulse while performing a vigorous exercise, try counting it immediately after the work-out. By counting the beats for 10 seconds and multiplying by six, you will have a relatively accurate estimate of your heart rate during exercise. With practice you will know how you feel when you reach your target heart rate and frequent checks will not be necessary.

The Exercise Session

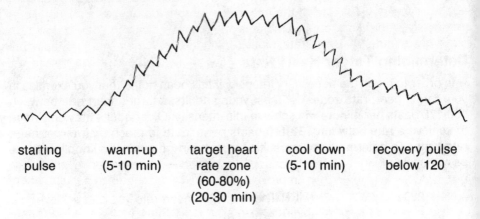

| starting pulse | warm-up (5-10 min) | target heart rate zone (60-80%) (20-30 min) | cool down (5-10 min) | recovery pulse below 120 |

The above diagram illustrates the typical pattern one should follow during each individual exercise session. It is important to develop the habit of including all steps — the elimination of any step, such as the cool-down, could lead to problems.

The Warm-up

The purpose of the warm-up phase is to prepare the body for the increased stress which will be placed upon it. If possible, the warm-up activity should relate specifically to the exercise to be performed. There are three important benefits to the warm-up session:

1.   The heart rate is gradually increased from the resting pulse.

2.   The temperature within the muscles is increased.

3.   Chances of muscle soreness and injury are lessened.

The Work-out

Guidelines for work-out sessions have been discussed previously. It is important to observe the principle of intensity and strive to reach the target heart rate.

The Cool-down

The cool-down allows the body to gradually return to its starting point. For this, simple slowing down of the exercise itself can be used. This gradual tapering is extremely important to prevent a possible pooling of blood in the lower extremities after vigorous endurance exercise. Without the contraction of the muscles in the extremities, the blood is not sent back to the heart and brain and may cause one to experience dizziness or faintness. In addition, light stretching assists in cooling the body and helps prevent soreness from unaccustomed use of muscles. This is also an excellent time to gain flexibility improvement.

The Recovery Heart Rate

One final check on the quality of any exercise session can be made by checking the recovery heart rate. If the intensity and duration of your work-out were appropriate, your heart rate five minutes after the exercise should be below 120 beats per minute. A heart rate higher than this indicates that perhaps the intensity of the program should be lowered and/or that the duration should be less. Remember your goal is to have an effective program but one that is not greatly uncomfortable — one that you can enjoy!

Training Guidelines

The basic purpose of any exercise program is to cause the body to improve — to adapt and adjust to the increased stress placed upon it. The body is a remarkable structure which is capable of adapting to stress and continually improving its efficiency. An improvement in physical condition results when exercise is increased in intensity and when an overload is presented to the body. One can overload the body by **increasing the resistance or work being done,** by **increasing the speed of the repetitions,** or by **increasing the number of repetitions.** Once the body adapts to this stress, the amount of work must be periodically increased in order for improvement to continue to occur. The progression should be gradual to prevent strain and soreness.

Another important consideration is the guideline of **specificity.** Improvement will best occur if the training program is specifically designed for that particular fitness component. For example, a strength program will develop strength, but one's cardiovascular endurance will best develop through participation in an aerobic exercise program. Select the exercise program which is appropriate for the specific fitness component sought.

And finally, it must be realized that no two people are alike. Everyone does not progress or improve at the same rate. Each person will respond to the training program in his or her own unique way and unique rate. Concentrate on the changes you are achieving and do not compare your progress with that of others. If you are observing the principles and guidelines noted in this chapter, you will eventually achieve your optimal level of fitness. Keep working but be patient!

REFERENCES

1. Fisher, A. Garth and Conlee, Robert K. *The Complete Book of Physical Fitness.* Brigham Young University Press, Utah, 1979.

2. Garrison, L; Leslie, P., and Blackmore, D. *Fitness and Figure Control.* Mayfield Publishing Co., Palo Alto, California, 1981.

3. Getchell, Bud. *Being Fit — A Personal Guide.* John Wiley & Sons, New York, 1982.

4. Golding, L., Myers, C., and Sinning, W. (eds.). *The Y's Way to Physical Fitness.* National Board of YMCA, Chicago, 1982.

5. Sharkey, Brian. *Physiology of Fitness.* Human Kinetics Pub., Champaign, Illinois, 1979.

6. U.S. Dept. of Health and Human Services. *Exercise and Your Heart.* U.S. Government Printing Office, Washington, D.C., 1981.

Chapter 4

FIND YOUR BEAT
■
Cardiovascular Fitness

In order to achieve an improved level of cardiovascular fitness, you must engage in a program of activities that will condition the heart, lungs, and vascular system. Vigorous exercises such as jogging, swimming, cycling, rope skipping, aerobic dance, and even walking are considered excellent choices for cardiovascular fitness.

In selecting your method for training the cardiovascular system make certain the activity meets the following guidelines:

1. the large muscle groups of the body (especially the hips and legs) are used

2. the activity can be sustained for at least 15-30 minutes

3. the activity is performed rhythmically (3)

Following are brief descriptions of basic exercise programs for improving your cardiovascular fitness. You may want to experiment with more than one program and utilize a variety to achieve your goal. Select the program which is enjoyable to you. Find your beat!

Walking

    I. Technique

        A. Remember walking for fitness is not the same as pleasure walking. No shuffling, strolling or sauntering is allowed!

        B. Concentrate on really using your muscles (and contracting them) — the feet, thighs, calves, buttocks, diaphragm, etc.

        C. Make certain you are in an upright position and that your entire foot is placed on the ground — heel first, then toes.

    II. **Procedure**

        A. Start slowly and use the first 3-5 minutes as a "warm-up." Increase your pace gradually.

        B. Try to get in rhythm with a natural, effortless motion.

C.   Use a stride that is natural for you but lengthen your stride gradually to increase the speed of your walking.

D.   As you quicken your pace, thrust harder with your legs, increase your arm swing, and breathe naturally.

III. **Suggested Program**

FITNESS CATEGORY = AVERAGE

Starter Walking Program (2)

Week	Frequency/Wk	Distance	Time
	Days	Miles	min:sec
1	3	2.0	34:16
2	3	2.0	34:16
3	3	2.0	30:00
4	4	2.0	30:00
5	3	2.5	37:50
6	3	2.5	37:50

Jogging

I. **Technique**

A.   Select comfortable, loose-fitting clothing (no plastic or rubberized clothing). Proper shoes are essential — those with well protected heel or arch support, firm soles, pliable tops, and proper fit.

B.   Run "tall" and keep your head up. Hold arms slightly away from the body and bend at the elbows.

C.   Either land first on the heel of the foot and rock forward to the ball of the foot or land on the entire bottom of the foot.

D.   Keep your steps short by letting the foot strike the ground beneath the knee.

E.   Breathe deeply while jogging. Breathe through your mouth and nose.

II. **Procedure**

A.   Begin slowly — perhaps a walking program is needed first.

B.   When starting, make certain you are comfortable and can talk with the person next to you.

C.   Pace yourself and stay at the same level for a longer period if it continues to challenge you.

III. **Suggested Program**

Running Program (start by walking, then walk and run, or run as necessary)

Under 30 years of age (2)

Week	Frequency/Wk	Distance	Time
		miles	min.
1	3	2.0	32:00
2	3	2.0	30:30
3	3	2.0	27:00
4	3	2.0	26:00
5	3	2.0	25:00
6	3	2.0	24:30
7	3	2.0	24:00
8	3	2.0	22:00
9	3	2.0	21:00
10	3	2.0	19:00
11	4	2.0	18:00
12	3	2.0 or	< 17:00
		2.5	< 22:00

Rope Skipping

I. **Technique**

A. Select a suitable rope: a #10 sash cord, commercial jump rope, or any piece of rope long enough to reach the armpits when held beneath the feet.

B. Use small circular movements of your arms; use mainly the hands and wrists.

C. Keep jumps small, spring mostly from the ankles, land as lightly as possible and allow just enough room for the rope to pass under your feet.

II. **Procedure**

A. Start with easy jumping from foot to foot as if running in place.

B. Next try jumping twice for every turn of the rope — once over the rope and then a small bounce while the rope passes overhead.

C. Try to keep your jumps continuous and jump only once for each turn of the rope.

D. Advance to hopping, running, kicking, rope crosses, and moving forward and backward.

E. If you tire too quickly, walk or jog slowly in place and then continue jumping.

III. **Suggested Program**

Week

1 - Jump 5 two-minute series (stretch between each series).

2 - Jump 5 three-minute series (stretch between each series).

3 - Jump 3 five-minute series with stretching.

4 - Jump 2 seven-minute series with stretching.

5 - Jump 10 minutes, stretch, then jump 5 minutes.

6 - Jump 15 minutes and stretch.

Cycling

I. **Technique**

A. Make certain the seat height is correct for you. Comfortable padding on the seat is a must for long rides!

B. Adjust the handle bars to a position which is comfortable for your riding style.

C. Pedaling must be vigorous and sustained to achieve real benefits.

D. Try to relax and enjoy the sights!

II. **Procedure**

A. Start with a moderate pace so your leg muscles can adjust gradually to the increased activity.

B. Remember it takes skill to safely handle a bike in traffic, on narrow roadways, and in tight situations. Learn how to handle your bike effectively before you attempt difficult situations such as heavy traffic or steep, winding roads. Be alert to holes or debris on the road.

C. Generally, you need to cycle twice as fast as you would jog to achieve your target heart rate (4). But in the beginning strive for a sustained ride and gradually increase your time or distance.

III. **Suggested Program**

Under 30 years years of age (2)

Week	Frequency/Wk	Distance	Time
1	3	2	9:00
2	3	2	8:00
3	3	3	10:45
4	4	3	10:00
5	4	4	15:00
6	4	4	14:30
7	4	5	18:30
8	4	5	18:00
9	5	5	17:30
10	4	6	22:30
11	4	6	22:00
12	4	6	21:30

Aqua Dynamics

I. **Technique**

A. Use these activities to improve not only cardiovascular endurance but to increase muscle tone, flexibility, calorie-burn-up, and release of tensions.

B. These activities are for the swimmer or the nonswimmer.

C. If possible, stay in water that is at shoulder level — the resistance of the water increases the strenuousness of your work-out.

II. **Procedure**

A. Swimmers can add lap swimming to their program. Choose a variety of strokes and make your work-out continuous. Change strokes as you need to. See the suggested starter program which follows.

B. Select a variety of exercises and perform them in a sequence that will keep your heart rate in the target zone.

C. Consider having music available and combining many of your aerobic dance steps with the usual water exercises.

III. **Suggested Program**

Swimming Program (overhand crawl) *

Under 30 years of age (2)

Week	Frequency/Wk	Distance	Time
		Yards	min.
1	4	300	12:00
2	4	300	10:30
3	4	300	10:15
4	5	500	20:00
5	5	500	18:00
6	5	500	17:00
7	5	200	4:00
8	5	300	6:00
9	5	400	8:00
10	5	500	10:30
11	5	600	12:30
12	4	800	15:30

* During the first 6 weeks, the goal is to swim the distance, but not necessarily continuously. Swim a distance that is comfortable, rest, then continue the swimming — resting cycle until the required distance is covered. Beginning with the seventh week, attempt to cover the distance without stopping.

Water Exercise Program

1. Walking (hands held up)
2. Jogging in place (2 min.)
3. Hopping — 1 and 2 legs
4. Toe Raising (or toe bounce)
5. STANDING WATER DRILLS

ARM EXERCISES:

Shoulders in the water
Palm up and down
Breast stroke
Circling

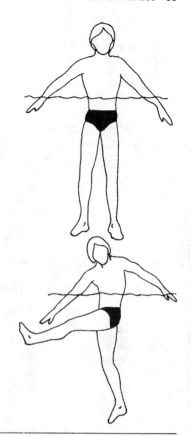

ALTERNATE TOE TOUCH

Standing, in waist-to chest-deep water, swimmer:

(1) Raises left leg bringing right hand toward left foot looking back and left hand extended rearward.
(2) Recover to starting position.
Repeat.
Reverse.

SIDE STRADDLE HOP

Stand in waist-to chest-deep water with hands on hips, swimmer:

(1) Jumps sideward to position with feet approximately two feet apart.
(2) Recovers.

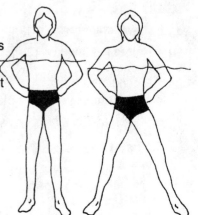

STRIDE HOP

Standing in waist-to chest-deep water with hands on hips, swimmer:

(1) Jumps, with left leg forward and right leg back.
(2) Jumps, changing to right leg forward and left leg back.
Repeat.

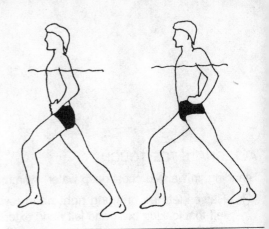

WALKING TWISTS

With fingers laced behind neck, swimmer:

(1) Walks forward bringing up alternate legs twisting body to touch knee with opposite elbow.
Repeat.

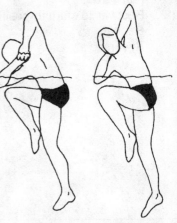

LEG OUT

Standing at side of pool with back against wall, swimmer:

(1) Raises left knee to chest.
(2) Extends left leg straight out.
(3) Stretches leg.
(4) Drops leg to starting position.
Repeat.
Reverse to right leg.

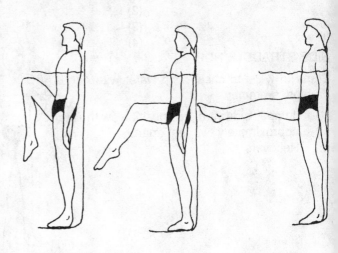

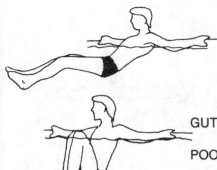

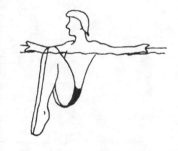

GUTTER-HOLDING DRILLS

POOL-SIDE KNEES UP

Supine, holding on to pool gutter with hands and legs extended, swimmer:

(1)   Brings knees to chin.
(2)   Recovers to the starting position.
      Repeat.

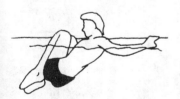

KNEES UP TWISTING

Supine, holding on to pool gutter with knees drawn up to chest, swimmer:

(1)   Twist slowly to left.
(2)   Recovers.
(3)   Twists slowly to right.
(4)   Recovers.
      Repeat.

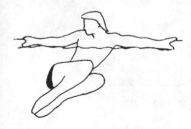

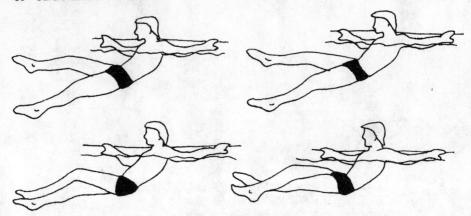

LEG CROSSES

Supine, holding on to pool gutter with legs extended, swimmer:

(1) Swings legs far apart.
(2) Brings legs together crossing left leg over right.
(3) Swings legs far apart.
(4) Brings legs together crossing right leg over left.
Repeat.

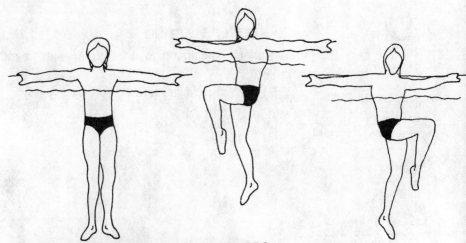

ALTERNATE RAISED KNEE CROSSOVERS

Standing, holding on to pool gutter with hands, back to wall:

(1) Lifts left knee and crosses it over. Twists to the right.
(2) Recovers.
(3) Lifts right knee and crosses it over, twisting to left.
(4) Recovers.

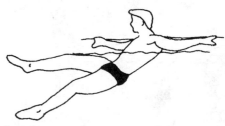

LEGS TOGETHER ON BACK

Supine, holding on to pool gutter with hands.
Legs together and extended with feet about 6''
under the water:

(1)   Spreads legs apart as far as possible.
(2)   Pulls feet and legs vigorously together.
      Repeat.

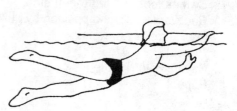

LEGS TOGETHER ON FRONT

Prone, holding on to pool gutter with one hand
flat on wall to push legs out, with feet together,
swimmer:

(1)   Spreads legs apart as far as possible.
(2)   Pulls feet and legs vigorously together.
      Repeat.

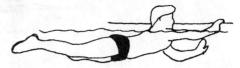

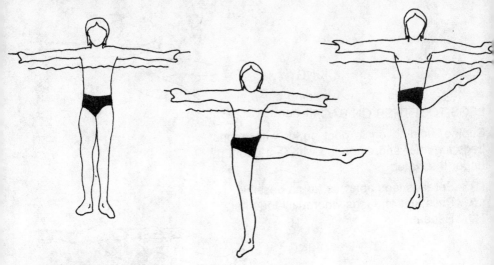

LEG SWING OUTWARD

Standing with back against poolside, and hands sideward holding gutter, swimmer:

(1) Raises left foot as high as possible with leg straight.
(2) Swings foot and leg to left side.
(3) Recovers to starting position by pulling left leg vigorously to right.
    Repeat.
    Reverses to right leg.
    Repeat.

BACK FLUTTER KICKING

Lying in a supine position and holding on to sides of pool with hand(s), swimmer:

(1) Flutter kicks.

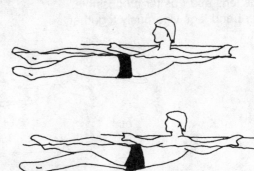

LEFT SIDE FLUTTER KICKING

Lying on a side position holding on to side of pool with right hand, with left hand braced on pool wall, swimmer:

(1) Flutter kicks.

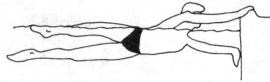

RIGHT SIDE FLUTTER KICKING

Lying on right side position, holding on to pool with left hand braced on pool wall, swimmer:

(1) Flutter kicks.

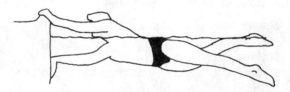

FRONT FLUTTER KICKING

Lying in a prone position holding on to side of pool with hand(s), swimmer:

(1) Kicks flutter style in which toes are pointed back, ankles are flexible, knee joint is loose but straight and the whole leg acts as a whip.

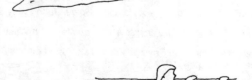

CLIMBING

Hands in pool gutter, facing pool side and feet flat against side and approximately 16'' apart, swimmer:

(1) Walks up side by approximately six short steps.
(2) Walks down the side to starting position. Repeat.

WITH KICK BOARDS

1   Flutter kick.
2. Side stroke.

WITH BALLS

1. Hold under water.
2. Basketball or keep away.

Aerobics

Dance right into the next chapter!

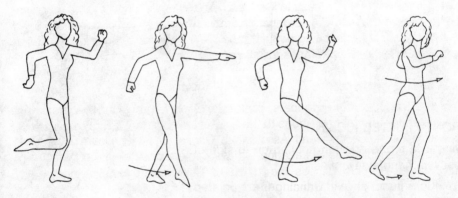

REFERENCES

1. Alexander, Ruth. *Focus on Fitness.* Maxwell King, Middleton, Kentucky, 1977.
2. Cooper, Kenneth. *The Aerobics Way.* Bantam Books, New York, 1977.
3. Fisher, A. Garth and Conlee, Robert K. *The Complete Book of Physical Fitness.* Brigham Young University Press, Utah, 1979.
4. Getchell, Bud. *Being Fit — A Personal Guide.* John Wiley & Sons, New York, 1982.
5. Getchell, Bud. *Physical Fitness: A Way of Life.* John Wiley & Sons, New York, 1976.
6. President's Council on Physical Fitness and Sports. *Aqua Dynamics.* U.S. Government Printing Office, Washington, 1977.
7. Vitale, Frank. *Individualized Fitness Programs.* Prentice-Hall Inc., Englewood Cliffs, New Jersey, 1973.
8. YMCA. *Physical Fitness Through Water Exercise.* National Board of YMCA, Rosemeont, Illinois, 1982.

Chapter 5

CATCH YOUR BEAT
■
Aerobic Dance

Discover

Catch the beat of a fun-filled, spirited, new style of dancing for fitness! Aerobic dancing is fast becoming a standard workout for cardiovascular conditioning as well as enhancing muscular endurance, flexibility, and graceful coordination. Most of the exercises are easy to learn and are the basis for enjoyable programs of fitness development. These dance-like exercise steps and patterns are set to the rhythmic beats of exciting popular music. This program is planned to satisfy the needs of all levels of fitness for all age groups.

Detect the Difference

Among the educators, dancers, professional performers, and organizations recognized for their contributions to the field of aerobic dance for fitness are the following: The American Heart Association, *Dance for Heart;* Joan Greggaens, television personality; Jack LaLanne, fitness centers and television personality; Mary Mayta, Aerobic Fitness Inc.; Richard Simmons, television personality; Jacki Sorensen, Aerobic Dancing Inc.; and the YMCA/YWCA.

In regard to aerobic dance classes, it is highly recommended that you investigate the credentials and instructional objectives of private dance studios, colleges, and community programs. Also check the qualifications and background credentials of their instructors. Styles may vary from one program to another. Many aerobic dancing classes are structured with organized materials and some are designed in free form. Both are suitable and some class sessions are based on both styles. What is important is that you decide the relative value of the particular styles in regard to your needs.

A sample dance routine has been designed as a dance lab (see Lab 15). You are invited to try this routine and use it three to four times consecutively. This routine will acquaint you with a structured style workout program. Later you may begin to develop and design other routines for your own special pace and needs. Once you are on your way to this free-style format, you may select your materials from the Digest of Terms (see the following pages). Although this format is free-style in its creativity and selectivity, you must remember to monitor the pace of your workout. Try to develop an approach that includes an acceleration, a plateau of the energy channel for your needs, stretching, and a deceleration to finish the program.

Design Your Workouts

1. Participate in regular class instruction.

2. Maintain a work level of 30 minutes to 1 hour and repeat three times weekly.

3. Practice and keep up with class material.

4. Dress appropriately.

   A. Wear comfortable clothing for exercise. (*Note:* No rubberized sweat pants or tops.)

   B. Choose good tennis or jogging shoes; must be light weight and flexible. (*Note:* No barefeet, stocking feet or ballet slippers.)

   C. Add a skip rope to your fitness wardrobe.

   D. A towel/exercise mat are optional, but worthwhile.

5. Learn to read your pulse accurately for the following times:

   A. Resting

   B. Warm-up

   C. Workout

   D. Recovery

   E. On floor exercise

   F. Cool-down

6. Take a pulse check:

   A. At the radial artery.

   B. Only for 6 seconds.

   C. Add a 0 (zero) to your pulse count.

   D. Assess your needs.

7. Pace your heart rate workouts. The heart must be gradually strengthened. The following suggestions permit you to increase your heart rate workouts at a safe pace. If necessary for your fitness condition start at:

   A. 120 beats per minute: Week 1-2

   B. Reach your minimum target heart rate level.

   C. Maximum Target Heart Rate: ongoing maintenance period after one month of class. (*Note:* Be aware of your breathing.)

8. Pace your fitness level.

   A. Warm-up (5-10 minutes)

   B. Workout - progress gradually (15-30 minutes)

   C. Interrupt your workouts with "interval stretching" times (30 sec.-1 min.)

   D. Intersperse workout and interval stretching times.

   E. Cool-down (5-10 minutes)

Distribute Your Effort

1. Acquire knowledge of fitness levels.

   A. Fitness is lost if workouts are less than two or three times weekly.

   B. Minimal workout time for each period is 30 minutes.

   C. Fitness is improved if workouts are three or four times weekly.

2. Recognize heart rate workouts.

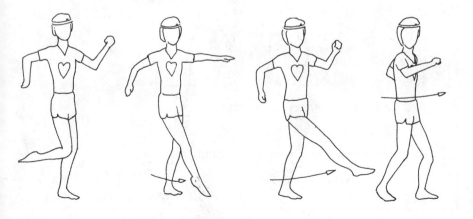

ANATOMICAL AWARENESS
(Bones)

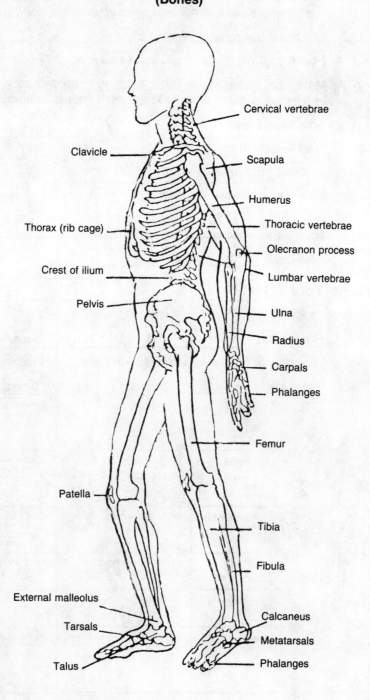

ANATOMICAL AWARENESS

(Muscles)

PART OF BODY	MAIN MUSCLES	APPROXIMATE LOCATION	MAIN MOVEMENT
ARMS AND SHOULDER	TRICEPS	Bottom of upper arm (when arm is lifted to side at right angle to body with palm up)	Straightens or extends elbow
	BICEPS	Top of upper arm (when arm is lifted to side at right angle to body with palm up)	Bends or flexes elbow
	PECTORALS	Front of chest	Rotate arm inward in shoulder socket and control some other arm movements
	TRAPEZIUS AND OTHER MUSCLES OF THE UPPER BACK	Upper back	Move scapulae (shoulder blades)
ABDOMEN	OBLIQUES	Over ribs on either side	Twists upper body to either side
	RECTUS ABDOMINIS	From upper ribs to top of pubic bone, covering abdomen area	Raises upper body forward as in sit-up
	QUADRATUS LUMBORUM	Small of back	1. Bends upper body to side 2. Stabilizes pelvis and spine
HIP AND UPPER LEG (THIGH)	GLUTEALS	Buttocks	1. Stabilize hip 2. Extend hip
	QUADRICEPS	Front of thigh	Extends leg in forward movements
	HAMSTRINGS	Back of upper leg	Bend knee
LOWER LEG	GASTROCNEMIUS (GASTROX OR CALF)	Back of lower leg	1. Points foot 2. *Raises* leg to ball of foot (half toe) 3. Bends knee
	SOLEUS	Back of lower leg under gastrox muscle	*Holds* leg in half-toe position (ball of foot)
	TIBIALIS AND PERONEUS	Around either side of ankle	Move ankle in circle
	ACHILLES TENDON	Lower part of leg and heel on back of leg; lower part of gastrox (calf) muscle	Same as gastrox

Adapted from *The Dancer Prepares: Modern Dance for Beginners,* 2e by James Penrodd and Janice Gudde Plastino by permission of Mayfield Publishing Company. Copyright © by Mayfield Publishing Company.

Determine the Facts

1.   Digest the terms

ABDOMINAL CRUNCHIE

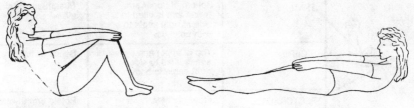

Bent-knee Crunchie   Long Line Crunchie

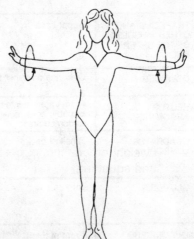

ARM CIRCLE

ARM FLING: May be performed standing or seated; keep arms parallel to the floor

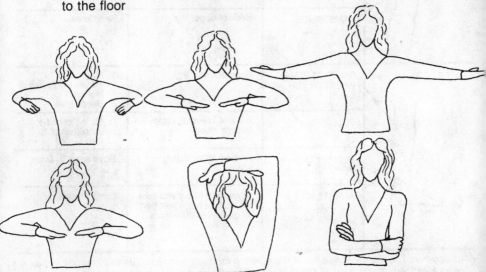

ARM WINDUP: Circling one or both arms in a 360 degree range from the shoulder

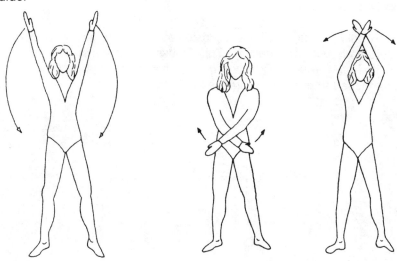

Á TERRE: Movement with weight on one foot or both feet on the ground (i.e., stepping, standing, and squatting)

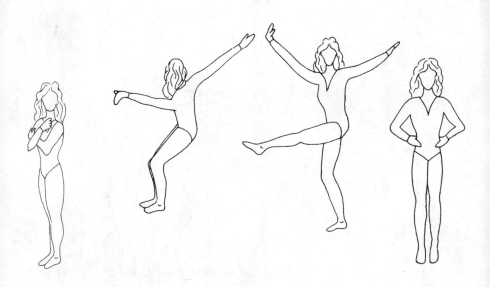

BARRE EXERCISES

BARRE: A pole or pipe designed for selected warm-up, skill development, drill, and cool-down activity. This fitness apparatus is designed horizontally to the workout floor and may be standing by portable supports or attached to a wall with braces for stationary use.

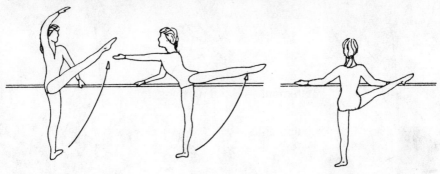

Work at the Barre

BATTEMENT: Leg kick to the side, front, or back of body line

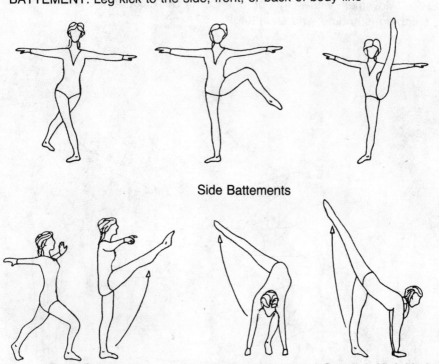

Side Battements

Front Battement   Side Lunge Variation   Swedish Kick Variation

BATTEMENT EN BAS: Work the free leg up and down; maintain a tight tummy.

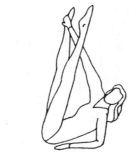

Battement — Seated Position

BEAT: The basic rhythmic pulse of the music or sound pattern

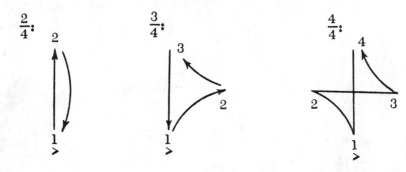

Examples: Jogging   Relaxation   Walking or Marching

BICYCLE

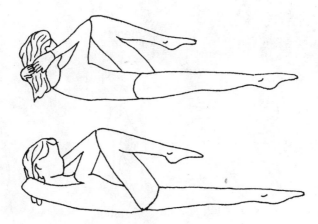

BODY ALIGNMENT: A proper balancing of body parts while standing or lying down. Create an imaginary plumb line passing through the side view perspective at the ear, shoulder, middle rib cage, center buttocks, back of knee, and to the front of ankle.

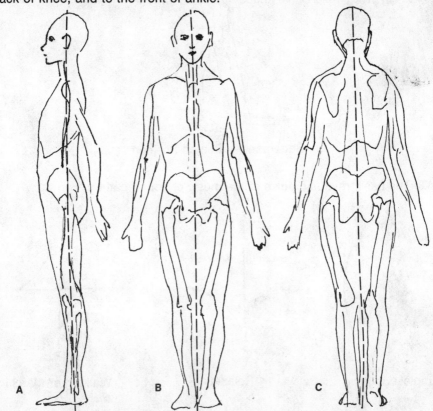

Normal postural alignment: A, Side view: **B**, Front view; **C**, Back view

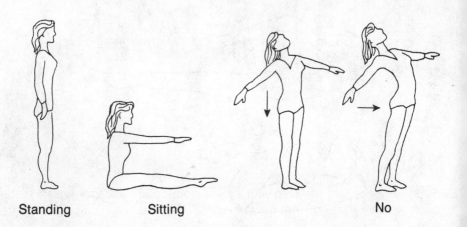

Standing   Sitting   No

BODY DROP SWING: perpendicular body swing from side to side or from high vertical to forward round-over and return. Movement must include a high to low level change and a waist hinge. NOTE: With side swings keep knees straight; with vertical drop swing move knees from a straight to bent to straight position.

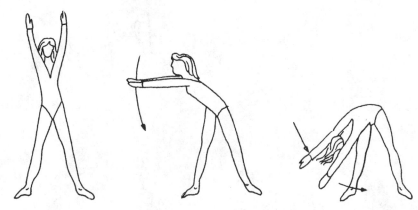

(1) Feet apart, arms to the ceiling   (2) Stretch right   (3) Sweep the floor

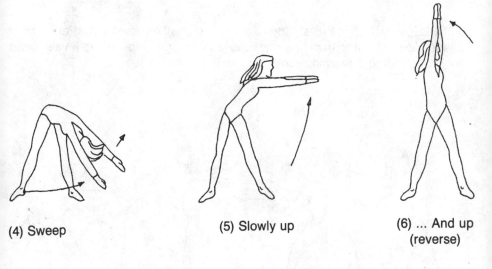

(4) Sweep   (5) Slowly up   (6) ... And up
                                                              (reverse)

BREAK: jump in place and clap with a lot of elbow; pull back energy as a follow-through from the clap; rhythm may be "slow" in 2 beats or "quick" in 1 beat.

"BUNS UP" — HIP-TORSO LIFT: Lie on back, bent knee position, arms along sides; raise hips, creating an oblique body line from knees to shoulders, then lower spine and hips; a repeatable movement.

Variation: Squeeze knees together while lifted.

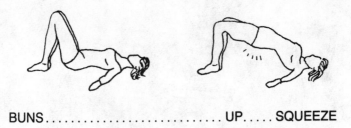

BUNS . . . . UP . . . . . SQUEEZE

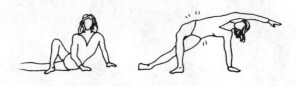

SIDE VARIATION

DOUBLE ARM SWING: Standing straddle leg position, swing both arms from side to side or front to back. As arms move from high to low to hip levels, bend the knees during the arm dropping movements.

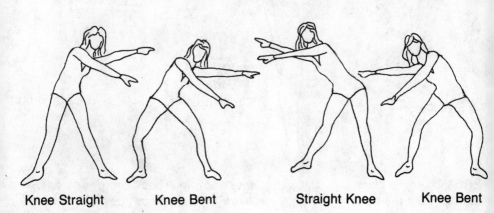

Knee Straight   Knee Bent   Straight Knee   Knee Bent

DYNAMIC DANCE ENERGY: refers to an ability to generate the force and flow of movement; an integral aspect in working at a meaningful energy level for desirable fitness gain.

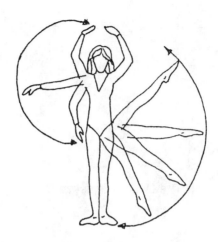

ECCENTRIC STEP AND/OR JUMP: movement sideward with heel-toe parallelism as weight is alternately exchanged from heel flips to toe flips; jumping heel-toe flips may be performed for more high-energy burn.

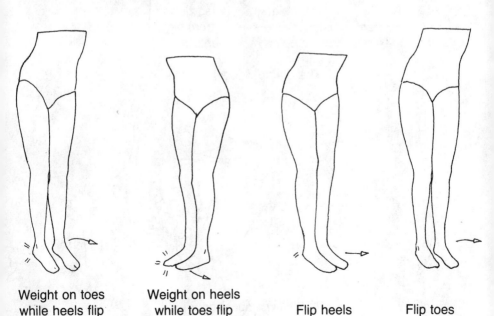

Weight on toes
while heels flip

Weight on heels
while toes flip

Flip heels

Flip toes

ELBOW SQUEEZES

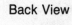

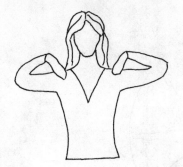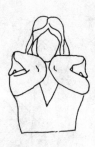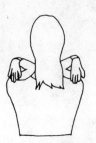

The Double Squeeze Cross

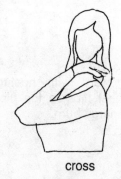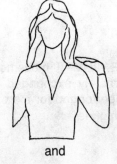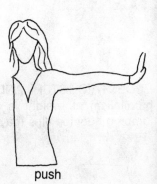

cross   and   push

The Single Squeeze Cross

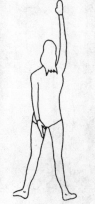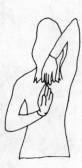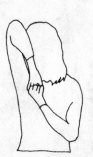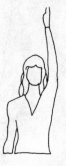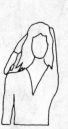

The Elbow Opposition

EN BAS: Movement is at a low level in relationship with the floor.

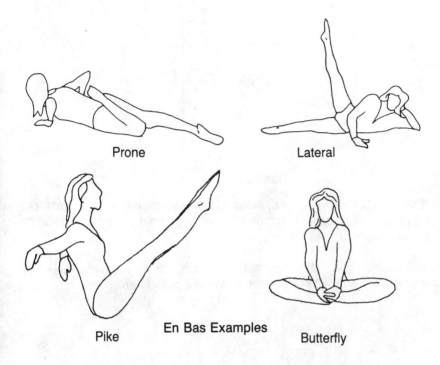

Prone

Lateral

Pike

En Bas Examples

Butterfly

EN L'AIR: Movement is at a high level in relationship to the floor.

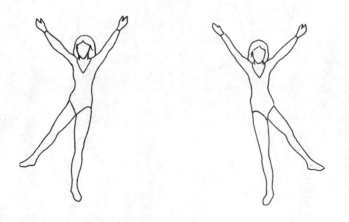

GRAND: Referring to a large range of movement in relationship to a dimensional size.

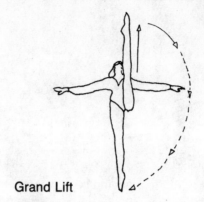

Grand Lift

GRAPEVINE STEP: Step to side, cross over next foot in front or in back of first foot; step sideward to same direction with first foot; hold weight on first and clap or snap; begin again to other side.

HOP SCOTCH: Jump straddle, hop in place, lifting opposite knee; jump straddle, hop in place with other foot, lifting opposite knee.

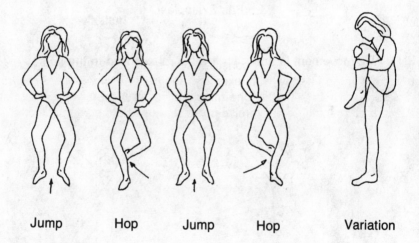

Jump   Hop   Jump   Hop   Variation

HOP WITH KNEE LIFT: Spring in the air from one foot while lifting the opposite knee either across the body line or in vertical position.

HURDLER'S QUAD STRETCH POSITION: Note caution to possible knee strain.

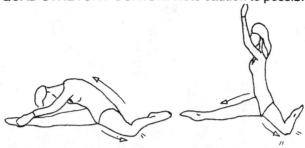

INCHWORM WALK OUT: From standing, bend forward to walk forward on hand-to-hand supports until body is in a bridge-like position to perform single or double heel lifts or rocks; return to standing position by either walking feet to hands or hands to feet and uncurling spine to a vertical standing position.

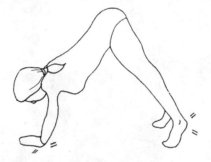

INTERVAL STRETCHING: A conscientious effort to perform a few stretching techniques intermittently with exercise and routine workouts. Perform such techniques for approximately one minute or for your preferred amount of time. Be aware of keeping your exercise pulse rate up. Hold static positions.

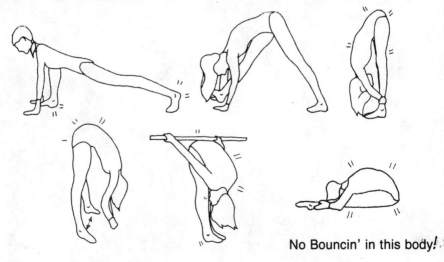

No Bouncin' in this body!

INTERVAL STRETCHING, *continued*

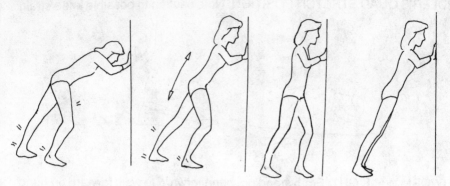

Work at the Wall

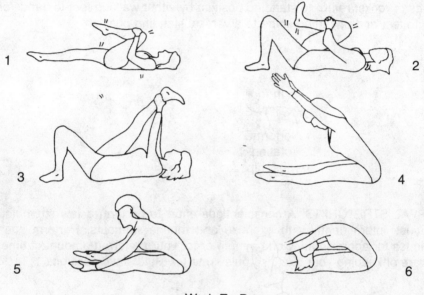

Work En Bas

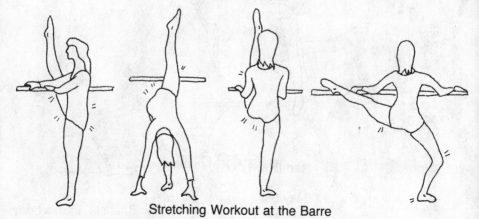

Stretching Workout at the Barre

INTERVAL STRETCHING, *continued*

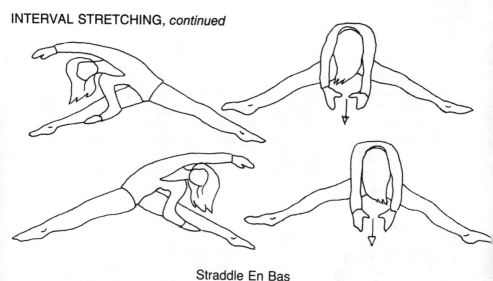

Straddle En Bas

IRISH ROCK: In-place jogging in a side-to-side or front-back position of feet; this may be a rope-skipping style in foot action also.

ISOLATIONS: Movements performed in directions going forward, backward, upward, downward and in rotation. Movement is applicable to various body parts; i.e., head, shoulders, ribs, hips and feet.

Head Rolls: Isolations

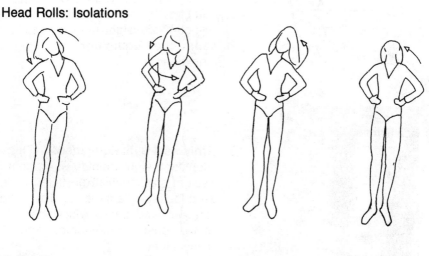

(1) Head Right   (2) Head Down   (3) Head Left   (4) Head Back

(May be reversed.)

Shoulder Isolations

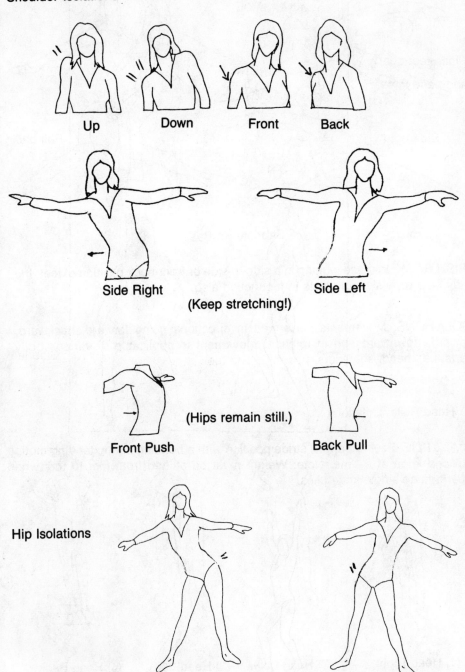

Up   Down   Front   Back

Side Right   Side Left

(Keep stretching!)

(Hips remain still.)

Front Push   Back Pull

Hip Isolations

Move at waist line and in hip sockets. Keep knees straight.

Hip Squares

Place feet apart
and bend knees.

Side right

Pull back

Push front

Side left

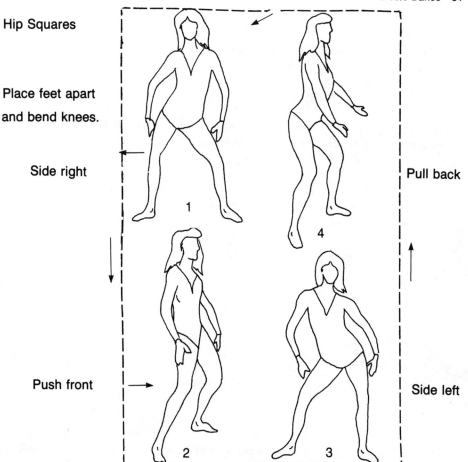

JAZZ PLIÉ: Feet in parallel stride position with a bending and extending motion in one knee at a time. Note: Weight must be shifted from foot to foot when performing single knee pliés.

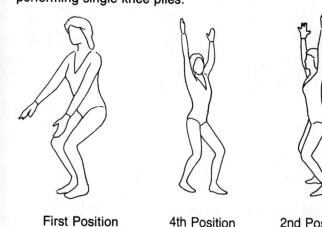

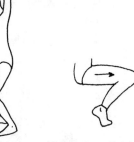

First Position   4th Position   2nd Position

Thigh parallel to floor
when heels are lifted

JOG A FIGURE EIGHT: Move in a jogging style while performing a figure eight floor pattern.

JOG A SQUARE: Creating a floor design of a square while jogging.

JOG HEEL SLAP: Jog in place while striking or touching the lifted heel in back with hand on same body side; step alternates.

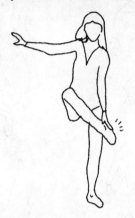

Heel Slap Opposition (Variation)

JUMP SNAP; JUMP CLAP: Syncopate the jump with snapping the fingers or clapping the hands; jumps may be performed in place, side to side, forward to backward or in a designed floor pattern.

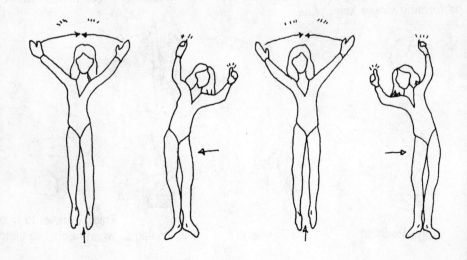

KNEE TO NOSE SWING

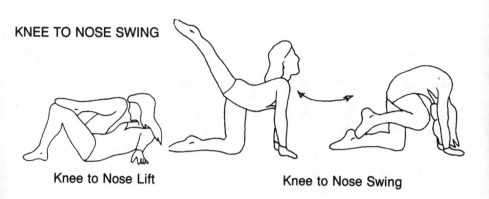

Knee to Nose Lift   Knee to Nose Swing

LEG SCISSORS

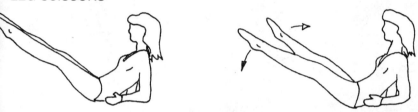

LEG SLICER SWING THRU: Lying on elbows on side or on back, swing as a slicing motion, a leg horizontally lifted from the floor; create own supports.

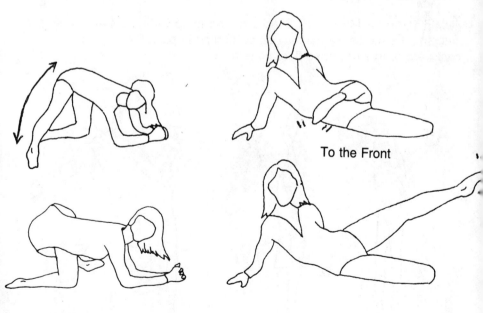

To the Front

On Elbows   To the Side

LET'S GET ON DOWN

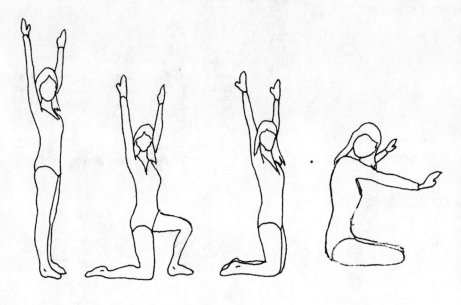

PATTERN 1

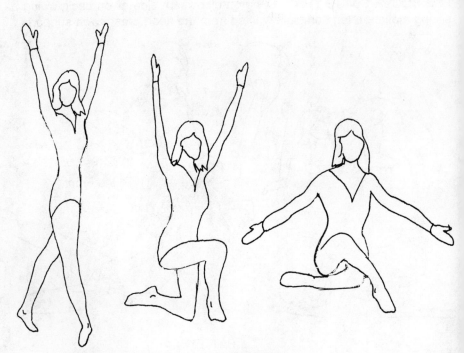

PATTERN 2

PATTERN 3

PATTERN 4

LET'S GET ON UP

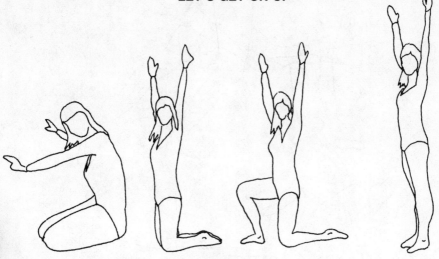

PATTERN 1

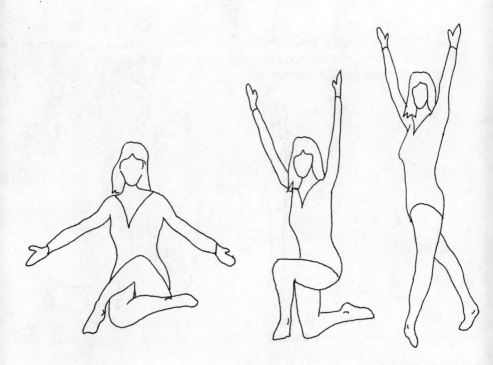

PATTERN 2

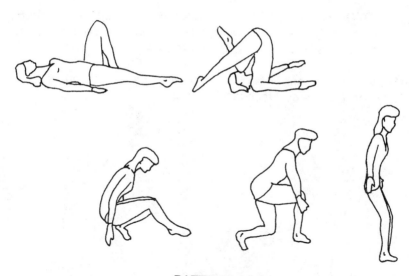

PATTERN 3

LOCOMOTOR MOVEMENT: (Walk, run, hop, jog, jump, pony step, pony two step, gallop, slide, skip and shuffle); spatial and temporal movement that travels from one standing base of support to the next.

LUNGE FORWARD, PULL-BACK AND CLAP: A fencer-style lunge forward or sideward and a rebound step, together with a clapping of hands during the step together; repeatable and/or alternating.

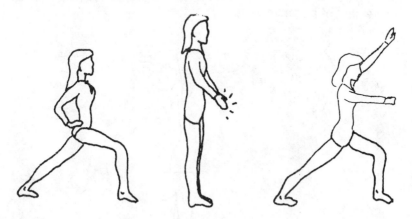

MUSICALITY: Your ability to create energy interpretation in your workout routines appropriate with the musical selections utilized.

MUSICAL TEMPO: The rate of speed and pace of the music; various tempos are useful for different energy level routines.

NONLOCOMOTOR MOVEMENT: (also referred to as Axial Movement); (Bend, stretch, rotate, upward, downward, twist, pivot and shake); basic movement that can be performed by a body part about its own axis.

OPPOSITION: A movement or body position with respect to normal opposing forces, body part useage or directionality.

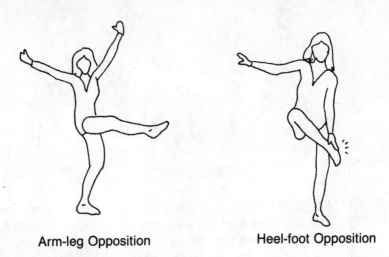

Arm-leg Opposition   Heel-foot Opposition

PETITE: Referring to a small range of movement in relationship to a dimensional size.

PLIE: The primary action of the knee and ankle area when performing the two-part movement of a bend and stretch of the leg.

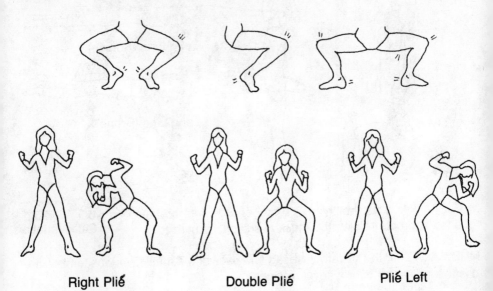

Right Plié   Double Plié   Plié Left

PONY TWO-STEP: A cha cha cha style pattern step performed side to side, forward to backward, or traveling.

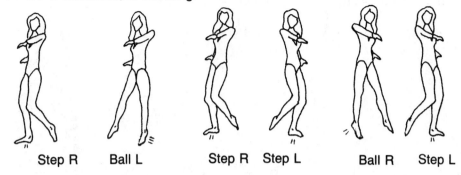

Step R   Ball L   Step R   Step L   Ball R   Step L

POSITIONS OF THE BODY: Several body positions relate to fitness workouts; maintain body alignment appropos to each: bent-knee, butterfly, long line, prone, side, straddle, supine, tuck, and yoga.

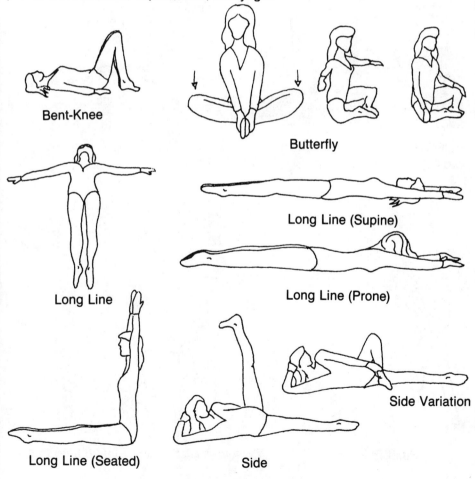

Bent-Knee

Butterfly

Long Line (Supine)

Long Line (Prone)

Long Line

Side Variation

Long Line (Seated)   Side

POSITIONS OF THE BODY, *continued*

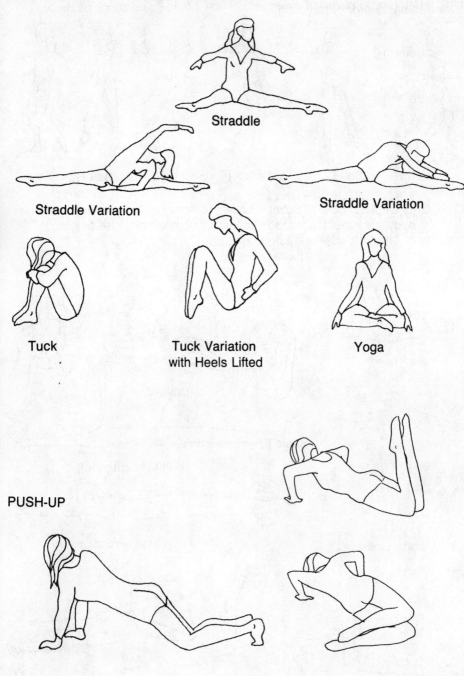

Straddle

Straddle Variation

Straddle Variation

Tuck

Tuck Variation
with Heels Lifted

Yoga

PUSH-UP

Modified Push-up

Push-up Variation with Side to Side Rolls

RHYTHM: The pulsation of a sequential flow of slow and quick beats or sounds.

Pattern 1 ___ Slow ___ Quick Quick ___ Slow ___ Quick Quick ___ Slow ___ Quick Quick

Pattern 2 Quick Quick ___ Slow ___ Quick Quick ___ Slow

RHYTHMIC SIT-UP: Touch toes, knees, roll down, roll up, elbow to lifted knee and repeat with other leg.

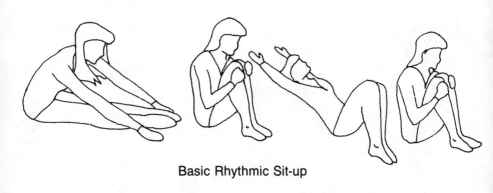

Basic Rhythmic Sit-up

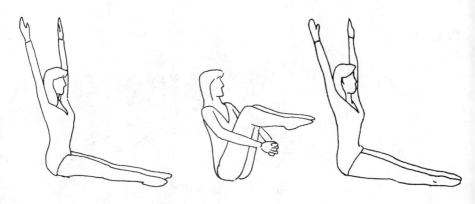

(add) Variation

ROCK AND PUNCH: In-place, straddle jogging while punching arms side to side, punching front right, front left and up and down.

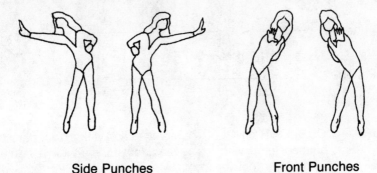

Side Punches   Front Punches

ROLLI-POLLI FOR HIPS: In bent line or long line leg positions, roll hips from side to side; create hand supports or arm coordinated swings.

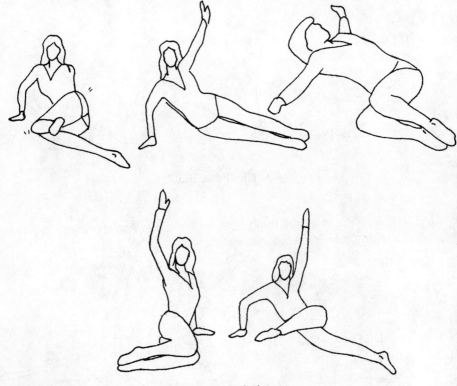

Rolli-Polli Variations

ROUTINE: Knowledge of a series of steps and patterns in an organized structure.

SEAT LIFT

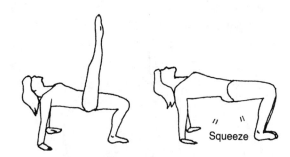

Squeeze

SCISSORS — DOUBLE OR SINGLE: A jumping action with a front-back position of feet; repeat bounce jump with same lead foot forward for a double, and continually exchange lead foot for a single step. *Variation:* Perform with side scissors and apart leg positions.

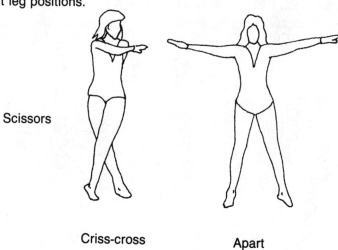

Scissors

Criss-cross

Apart

SQUAT WALK: Walk in a bent thigh position while planting the whole foot flatly with each walking step (forward, backward, sideward).

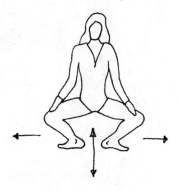

STRETCH-UP (Also labeled reaches): Side to side stepping in place, while performing rib stretches with arms held above the head.

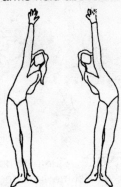

SUPINE LEG CIRCLE: May be performed by one leg or both legs.

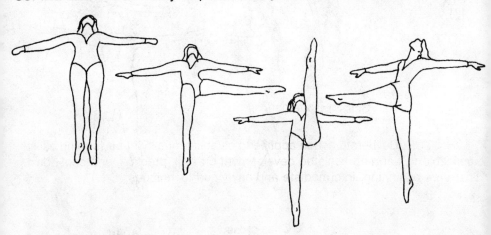

SWEDISH LUNGE KICK

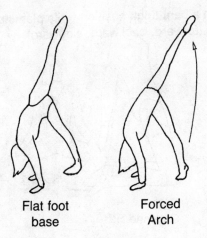

Flat foot
base

Forced
Arch

TABLE TOP POSITION: Standing in a forward waist bend position while maintaining a horizontal line to the floor from the spine to the head; create your own stance.

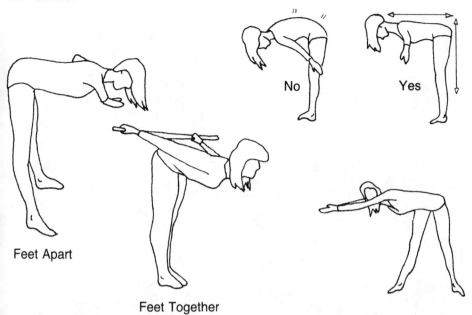

No   Yes

Feet Apart

Feet Together

TECHNIQUE: Deliberate action applied to establish quality in performing skills; applicable to warm-up, isolated development on skill, practice, and cool-down. There are beginning, intermediate and advanced techniques.

THIGH-LEAN OBLIQUE

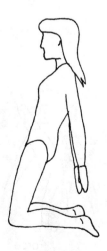

On Knee Base

THIGH LIFT

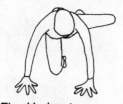

Fire Hydrant
(Extend from knee)

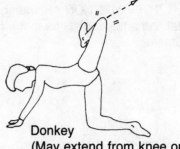

Donkey
(May extend from knee or
lift and lower thigh)

INNER THIGH LIFTS: Lie on side of body, cross upper leg over underneath leg, support on elbow, raise and lower vertically the underneath leg.

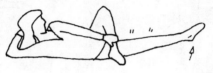

OUTER THIGH LIFT

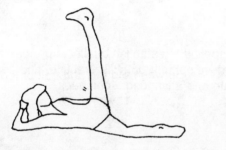

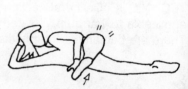

WAIST TWIST: May be performed with straight legs, in plié; or variations on the floor.

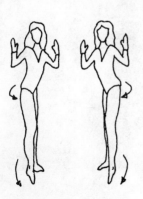

Variation 1

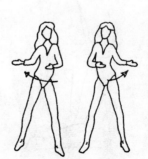

Variation 2

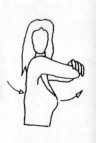

Variation 3

WAIST TWIST, *continued*

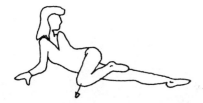

Variation 4

WEIGHT DISTRIBUTION ON THE FEET

                    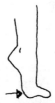

Standing on flat foot   Between big toe and ball of foot

WINDMILL

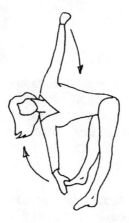

Use Opposition and Torque

2. Practice:

   A. Warm-ups

   B. Work-outs

   C. Interval Stretching

   D. Cool-downs

3. Drill and practice patterns and step combinations.

4. Design a free-style program by randomly selecting a good choice of steps and patterns based upon the Digest of Terms. *Note*: Choose with practical knowledge and counseling from your instructor.

5. Perform a variety of dancing, aerobic-style routines and designed programs. (See Dance Lab as suggested sample workout.)

6. Concentrate on your self-control.

7. Energize yourself! Plug in your unit!

8. Select some up-beat popular musical scores to let your spirits rise! Following is a brief list of suggestions to help get you started on your record library: *Fame* album, *Planet Rock* album, *Hooked on Classics* album, Disco sounds, Country-Western music, Broadway show tunes, Herb Alpert scores, Henri Mancini scores.

   These and almost any musical arrangement can be adapted to aerobic dance and exercise routines. Go for it!

9. Drink plenty of liquids.

10. Establish a nutritionally well-balanced diet.

Decide to Go For It!

Grab the beat!

The word *aerobic* means "with oxygen." Its reference to fitness programs in aerobic training was directly the result of research conducted by Dr. Kenneth Cooper, who developed a fitness program in the early 1960's with the Air Force. He studied the benefits of oxygen uptake created by designed exercise tests. He concluded that any exercise which increased the heartbeat to an exercise workout rate during an interval of sustained time created an improvement in cardiovascular health.

Dance movements for aerobic dancing are designed to create combinations of steps and patterns utilizing space, and the elements of time and dynamics. There must be an ebb-flow exchange of energy. Furthermore, self-control and concentration must be maintained. Musicality is exhibited by the performance of the harmony between the outlet of positive energy and the sensitivity of feeling free and having a wonderful time!

Join in to a fitness style program which will improve your body's efficiency, increase your resistance to fatigue, assist you with weight control, make you look great and feel so good!

Catch your beat!

REFERENCES

1. Lockhart, Aileene S. and Pease, Esther E. *Modern Dance: Building and Teaching Lessons.* Wm. C. Brown Co., Dubuque, Iowa, 1982.

2. Loren, Teri. *The Dancer's Companion: The Indispensable Guide to Getting the Most Out of Dance Classes.* Dial, New York, 1978.

3. Mata, Mary. *Aerobic Fitness.* Hoctor Products for Education, Waldwick, New Jersey, 1982.

4. Missett, Judi and Meilach, Dona Z. *Jazzercise: Rhythmic Jazz Dance — Exercise.* Bantam, New York, 1978.

5. Nochollds, Bronwen. *Move!* Plays, Boston, 1975.

6. Penrod, James and Plastino, Janice Gudde. *The Dancer Prepares: Modern Dance for Beginners.* Mayfield Publishing Co., Palo Alto, California, 1980.

7. Sherbon, Elizabeth. *On the Count of One: Modern Dance Methods.* Mayfield Publishing Co., Palo Alto, California, 1975.

8. Shyne, Kevin. *Dance for Your Life!* Reader's Digest, Pleasantville, New York, April, 1982.

Chapter 6

STRETCH OUT AND SHAPE UP
■
Flexibility Fitness

What?

Although flexibility can be defined in many ways, a definition must include the essence of one's ability to be resilient and pliable. In short, flexibility is the range of motion the body joints can move through. Each person's musculature and joint structure is different; one person may have a lighter or heavier skeletal structure than another and may or may not be able to move through a full range of flexibility movement.

Many exercises may be used for light stretching or serious stretching to improve one's flexibility fitness level. Several warm-up and cool-down stretching exercises are provided in this chapter to acquaint you with a varied program of flexibility exercises.

What About the Warm-Up?

It is important to begin each workout with a few minutes of warm-up exercises to circulate blood to your muscles and to increase your heart rate.

1. **Warm-Up** with **light quick activity; 1-3 minutes** (i.e., in-place marching, toe-heel pedalling in place, light jogging or/and light jumping jacks).

2. **Warm-Up** with **static stretching: 3-8 minutes** (i.e., refer to Interval Stretching in Chapter 6, preferably seated).

3. **Mentally** prepare yourself with enthusiasm for a good workout.

When you warm-up or cool-down you must use the body's principal joints and move them through a full working range of motion. It cannot be emphasized too strongly that the flexibility warm-up and cool-down exercises are important to your total workout and will help you feel better.

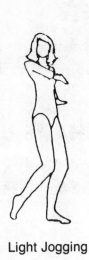

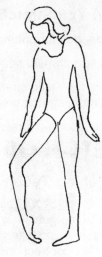

Light Jogging   Toe-Heel
                                 Pedalling

WARM-UP

What About a Bouncing or Ballistic Stretch?

The bouncing stretch is one way of stretching but it is not the best way. Sometimes called dynamic or ballistic stretching, this particular kind of movement may stimulate a stretch reflex and inhibit the muscle which needs to be stretched from properly stretching out. Ballistic stretching has a bouncy, bobbing-like motion and can easily cause a muscle tear and extreme soreness. It is advisable to avoid this technique.

A better type of stretch is the **static** stretching technique. This is the method recommended for flexibility exercise. To perform static stretching do the following:

1. Use proper alignment; important for your body position.

2. Stretch **slowly** and concentrate on what you are feeling in the position and stretch.

3. Hold your muscles in your stretch position for 10-20 slow counts (seconds).

4. Stretch to the point of feeling tightness.

5. Release the tightness slowly after you have counted and held your position.

6. When necessary gently shake out the tightness.

7. Move immediately to the next stretch position.

This static stretching technique allows the muscle fibers to relax and to counteract the stretch reflex built into your body.

What to Do When You Stretch?

1. Try to stretch every day for optimal fitness.

2. Begin your static stretch held positions from 10-20 seconds.

3. Gradually increase the static stretch hold to 30 seconds, to 40 seconds, to one minute (maximum stretch time for each position).

4. Be sure to include warm-up stretches before each workout.

5. Conclude with cool-down stretches after each workout.

Variation in Stretching Technique?

Facilitation of the proprioceptors is a term applied to a physiological action in which a contraction of a muscle is normally concluded by the sequential relaxation of that muscle's opposite antagonistic muscle. While in a stretched position, one may forcibly contract one muscle group against a resistance. After holding the contraction for 6 to 10 seconds, immediately begin to carefully let go and gradually stretch what was being contracted. This is a proprioceptive muscular facilitation; it allows the gradual stretching of an opposing set of muscles to work from the resisting set of muscles that were held in contraction.

The method of proprioceptive muscular facilitation is as follows:

1. Use proper alignment and position readiness.

2. Concentrate on feeling the movement.

3. Contract.

4. Release (gently let go).

5. Stretch to tightness again.

6. Repeat 3 more times.

What Are Some Static Stretches?

The following flexibility exercises are referred to as static stretching techniques and are the recommended types of stretching that should be performed for best results.

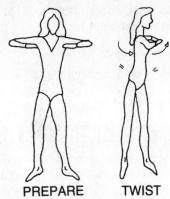

PREPARE   TWIST

1. Standing Waist Twist

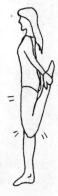
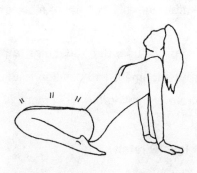

2. Quad Stretch

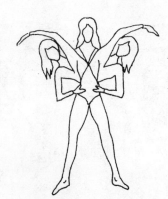

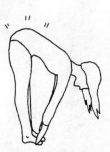
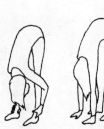

TOE TOUCH   VARIATION OF FEET

3. Side Bend Stretch   **4. Toe Touch Stretch**

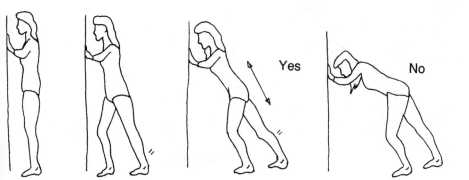

5. Achilles and Calf Stretch

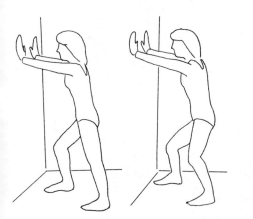

6. Soleus Stretch

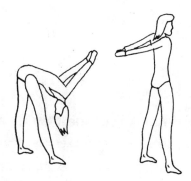

7. Armpit Stretch
Caution: Do not over-stretch!

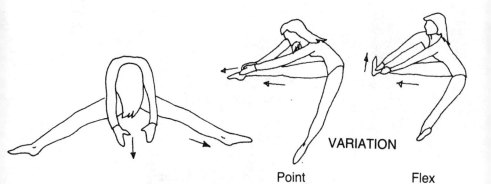

8. Straddle Sit Stretch
(Variation to each leg)

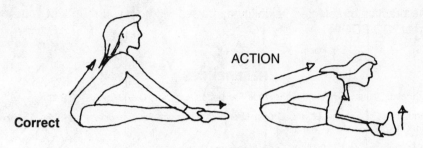

Correct

ACTION

9. Long Line Sit Stretch

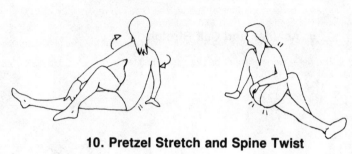

10. Pretzel Stretch and Spine Twist

What About the Cool-Down?

The cool-down exercises should complete your workout.

1. **Repeat** several **static stretches** of 5-8 minutes.

2. Slip into warm-up jacket or suit to keep your muscles warm.

3. Allow for a gradual reduction of your heart beat and taper off slowly.

4. After five minutes' rest, your pulse should be under 120 beats per minute. The pulse rate should be under 100 beats per minute after 10 minutes.

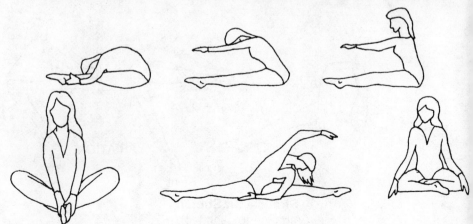

The practice of selected flexibility exercises will help you roundout your total workout. GO FOR IT!

REFERENCES

1. Arnheim, Daniel D. *Dance Injuries: Their Prevention and Care.* C. V. Mosby Co., St. Louis, 1975.

2. Morehouse, Laurence E. and Gross, Leonard. *Maximum Performance.* Pocket Books, New York, 1977.

3. Mott, Jane A. *Conditioning and Basic Movement Concepts.* Wm. C. Brown Co., Dubuque, Iowa, 1968.

4. Penrod, James and Plastino, Janice Gudde. *The Dancer Prepares: Modern Dance for Beginners.* Mayfield Publishing Co., Palo Alto, California, 1980.

5. Sheffield, Emilyn A. *Total Fitness for Women.* Goodyear, Santa Monica, California, 1980.

6. Sherbon, Elizabeth. *On the Count of One: Modern Dance Methods.* Mayfield Publishing Co., Palo Alto, California, 1975.

Chapter 7

GET PHYSICAL
■

Muscular Fitness:
Strength and Endurance

WHY?

Basic to any discussion of improving strength and endurance fitness is an understanding of the value and benefits to be gained from the program. Many people, especially women, feel that since they are not interested in developing larger muscles (body building), there is no need for strength training. However, such an opinion overlooks the tremendous advantages when we achieve an appropriate level of muscular strength and endurance.

There is ample evidence that stronger muscles better protect the joints which they cross, making one less prone to joint injuries. Muscles with greater strength and endurance are also less susceptible to strains, sprains, and pulls. Another important benefit is that better tone in the muscles of the trunk aids in preventing some of the common postural problems such as low back pain, round shoulders, and sagging abdominals. Additional reasons for maintaining an adequate level of strength and endurance are to enhance one's performance in sports, to make one less susceptible to fatigue, to aid in the rehabilitation of injured muscles, and to help one look and feel better. As people improve their body appearance by firming muscles and developing a better shape, their self-concept and outlook on life usually improve.

In order to develop better strength fitness, each individual must first assess his or her own particular level of strength and endurance. The selected tests in Chapter 2 provide information about the areas in greatest need of improvement. The specific goal you wish to attain will determine the type of exercise program which will produce the best results. Knowing the correct procedures for effective strength training will lead to faster rates of improvement and fewer injuries. In addition, the potential for achieving muscle size and strength is largely determined by genetic makeup. This is why women do not develop large bulging muscles when involved in a weight training program. Females generally have about one-third fewer muscle fibers than men and the male hormone, testosterone, contributes to muscle growth and hypertrophy. However, an individualized program for strength and muscular fitness can help every person to improve.

How?

The basic ingredient of a muscular fitness training program is progressive resistance of the muscle. The goal is to single out a specific muscle group and gradually apply greater and greater stress to it. A high intensity program (heavier weights or resistance) with fewer repetitions will specifically lead to gains in muscle strength. A low intensity (lighter weights or using one's body weight) with many repetitions (20 or more) will lead to gains in muscular endurance. In either program it is important to gradually increase the intensity of the workout so that the muscles will respond positively and not suffer extreme tissue damage. All of the principles and guidelines for training discussed in Chapter 3 should be observed as one participates in a muscular fitness program.

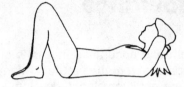

1. **Natural Resistance** — your own body weight, manual resistance from a partner, and/or isometric exercises.

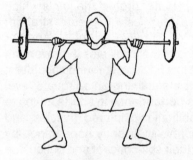

2. **Barbells and Dumbbells** — Commonly referred to as free weights, these can be utilized in a variety of ways. Barbells are designed for two-handed lifts and dumbbells for one-handed lifts. The amount of weight used may be varied and the equipment is relatively inexpensive.

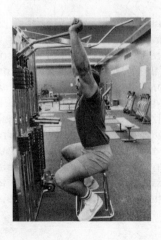

3. **Universal Gym Equipment** — This very popular weight training equipment has weight stacks which are lifted by lever and pulley attachments. The weights are on fixed tracks which make them safe, easily adjustable, and very convenient.

4. **Nautilus Equipment** — This equipment uses a cam system to provide resistance that changes to match the joint's ability to produce force throughout the range of motion and an accommodating resistance device.

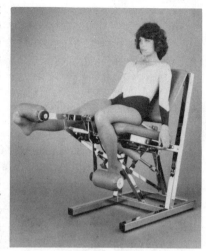

5. **Mini-Gym and Hydra-Gym Equipment** — Training devices that automatically vary the resistance in response to the amount of muscular force applied. This equipment enables one to perform exercises at a variety of speeds with maximum resistance.

Where?

For individuals interested in learning more about the various types of weight training equipment and in learning how to establish a specific program, it is best to investigate one or more of the many outstanding publications listed below. These sources are very comprehensive and will give a more complete description of the exercises which can be performed.

Weight Training Everyone by Rich Tuten, Clancy Moore and Virgil Knight. Winston-Salem, N.C.: Hunter Textbooks Inc., 1982.

Strength Fitness: Physiological Principles and Training Techniques by Wayne Westcott. Boston: Allyn & Bacon, 1982.

Strength Training Principles by Ellington Darden. Winter Park, Fla.: Anna Publishing Co., 1977.

Ready, Set, Go!

As previously stated, it is quite possible to develop muscular fitness by using the natural resistance of your own body weight to help you. The following exercises are designed to be done at home or at school; all that is needed is a clear area of floor and possibly an exercise mat or padded carpet for comfort. Remember to warm up before starting and cool down when you finish. Start slowly with a few repetitions and increase the intensity as you progress. Many of these exercises are especially beneficial in improving muscular endurance.

ABDOMINALS

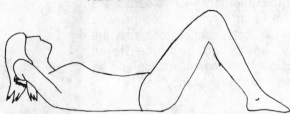

BASIC CURL UP: Curl straight, twist to left, twist to right, and twist bringing opposite knee to elbow.

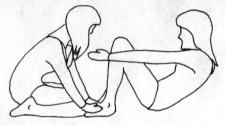
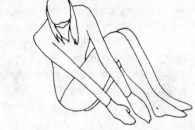

Curl up with arms extended to side of knees. Hold.

Curl up with arms extended on outside of knees. Hold.

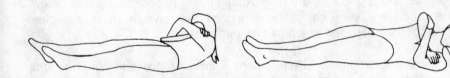

Curl head and shoulders and twist to the side.   Hold.

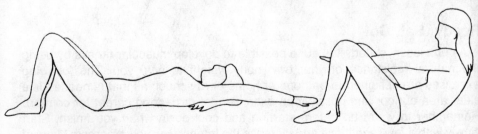

Raise head slowly and hold.

ABDOMINALS

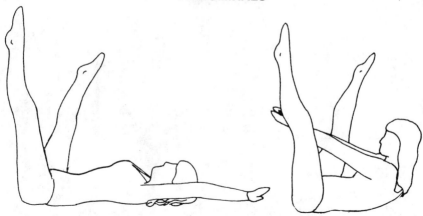

Curl to a sit-up position with arms between legs.
Hold.

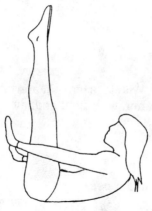

Curl to the sit-up position with arms extended,
wrists flexed, palms out and push with arms.

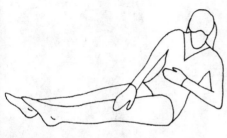

Curl up with one arm extended to
outside of opposite leg. Hold.

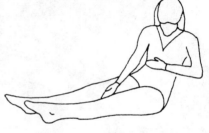

Curl up with one arm extended to inside
of opposite leg. Hold.

ABDOMINALS

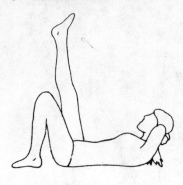

Leg extended, toes pointed, raise to a sit-up position reaching for toe.

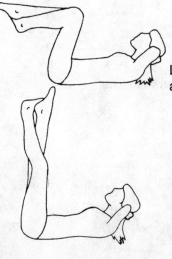

Lift feet off floor with knees bent and cross legs at ankles. Curl up and twist to the right and left.

With legs straight and crossed at knees, curl up and twist right and left.

ELEVATED LEG CURLS: Roll head, neck, and shoulders and hold.

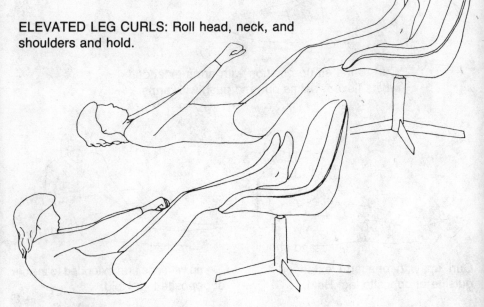

TRICEPS

Chair push-up

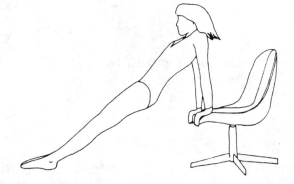

TRICEP PRESS: Lift until arms are straight and
hold. Lower slowly back to the floor.

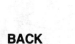

BACK

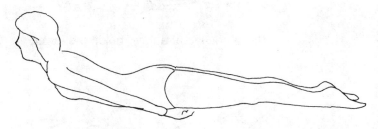

Lift head and shoulders off floor. Hold.

BACK

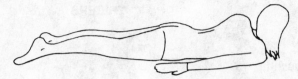

Lift head and shoulders and twist to the side. Hold.

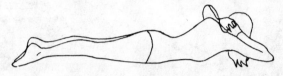

Hands behind head. Lift head and shoulders twisting to the side. Hold.

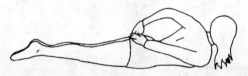

Hands behind back. Lift head and shoulders twisting to the side. Hold.

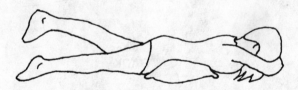

Raise one leg at a time, hold, and lower.

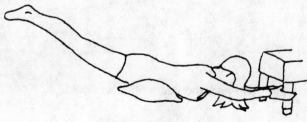

Raise both legs at a time.

LEGS

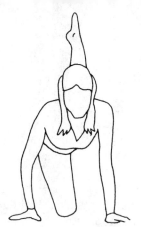

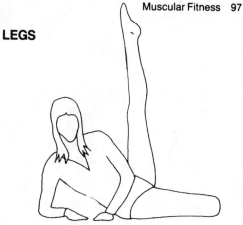

Extend leg straight; raise and lower — foot flexed and then pointed.

Raise and lower leg — foot flexed, then pointed, then flexed.

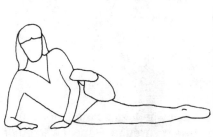

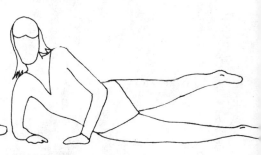

Extend leg to front of body. Raise and lower leg — foot flexed, then pointed, then flexed.

Swing leg from just behind other foot to as far in front as possible.

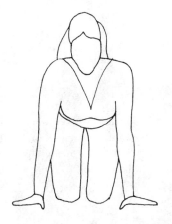

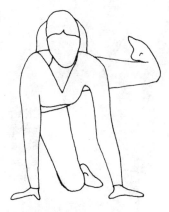

Raise and lower leg to the side.

LEGS

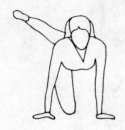

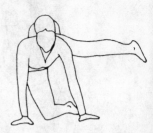

Swing leg forward and back.

With leg extended to the side, foot flexed, circle forward with your foot.

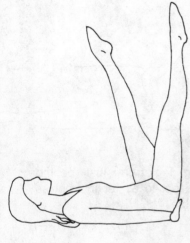

Lift leg in front with toes pointed, flex foot, point toes and lower to ground. Repeat with other leg. Repeat with both legs together. *Variation:* Lift right leg with pointed foot and quickly change legs in air.

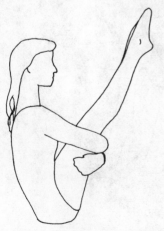

Bring knees to chest and hold with arms. Extend leg as straight as possible; lower to beginning. Repeat with other leg and then repeat with both legs at once. Do not allow back to sink as legs extend.

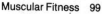

OUTER THIGH

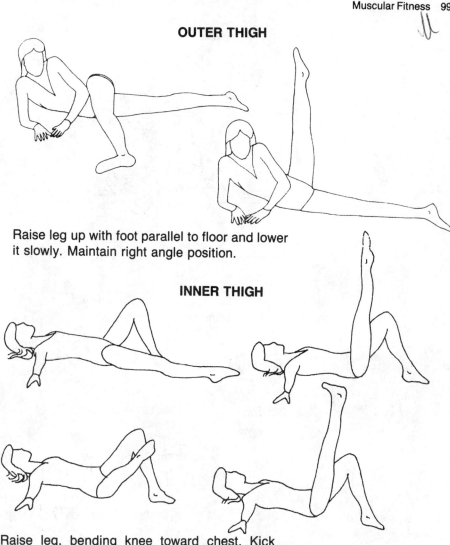

Raise leg up with foot parallel to floor and lower it slowly. Maintain right angle position.

INNER THIGH

Raise leg, bending knee toward chest. Kick straight up pointing toe to ceiling. Slowly lower to side keeping toe pointed until about 10 inches from floor. Flex foot, raise and lower leg.

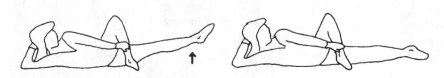

Raise extended leg and hold. Foot extended and then flexed.

HIPS

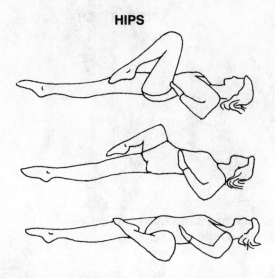

Keep shoulders on floor and foot in place as you swing knee as far to the side as possible.

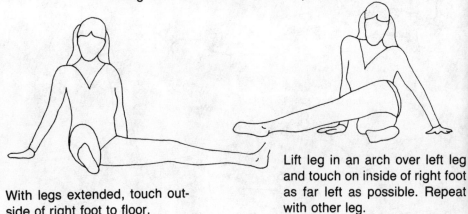

With legs extended, touch outside of right foot to floor.

Lift leg in an arch over left leg and touch on inside of right foot as far left as possible. Repeat with other leg.

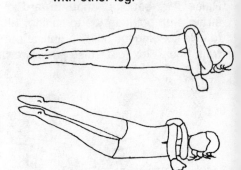

Bend knee and raise leg as high as possible. Hold.

Raise top leg, bring lower leg up. Hold.

PARTNER RESISTANCE

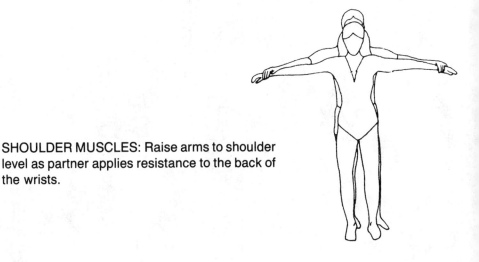

SHOULDER MUSCLES: Raise arms to shoulder level as partner applies resistance to the back of the wrists.

OUTSIDE OF THIGH: Raise leg as high as possible with resistance to side of leg.

SHOULDER: Raise arm as resistance is applied to back of hand.

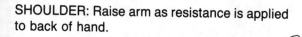

PARTNER RESISTANCE

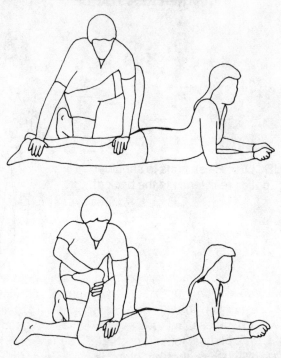

HAMSTRING CURL: Raise leg with toes pointed toward knee. Raise as high as possible, hold, and return slowly to ground. Resist at the heel and leg.

REFERENCES

1. Baley, James. *Illustrated Guide to Developing Strength, Power, and Agility.* Parker Publishing Co. Inc., West Nyack, New York, 1977.

2. Darden, Ellington. *Especially for Women.* Leisure Press, West Point, New York, 1977.

3. Riley, Daniel. *Maximum Muscular Fitness.* Leisure Press, West Point, New York, 1982.

4. Sheffield, Emilyn. *Total Fitness for Women.* Goodyear Publishing Co., Santa Monica, California, 1980.

5. Tuten, Rich; Moore, Clancy; and Knight, Virgil. *Weight Training Everyone.* Hunter Textbooks Inc., Winston-Salem, N.C., 1982.

6. Westcott, Wayne. *Strength Fitness.* Allyn & Bacon, Inc. Boston, 1982.

Chapter 8

FOOD FOR THOUGHT
■
The Role of Nutrition

If you are truly serious about achieving a high level of personal fitness, then it is imperative that you not only understand the role of nutrition but apply the principles of proper nutrition to your daily eating plan. To train and condition hard to improve your fitness but neglect the rules of good nutrition is to automatically limit the potential for improvement. You can only hope to achieve your optimal level of fitness through a combined program of well-planned exercise and attention to the fundamentals of good nutrition. Actually, proper nutrition forms the foundation for physical performance. It provides the fuel for our work and the elements for utilizing the potential energy contained within this fuel. Perhaps the importance of understanding nutrition is best stated by Dr. Jean Mayer, one of the country's most respected nutritionists: "Most of our major causes of death and disability — heart disease and stroke, high blood pressure, adult onset diabetes, liver and kidney diseases — either result from faulty nutrition or from a combination of factors that include poor nutrition . . . A few simple changes in the American diet and habits of life could greatly reduce the number of people who acquire these diseases and who may die from them."

One of the problems which prevents changes in eating habits is the number of myths, distortions and actual fallacies surrounding the area of nutrition.

It is difficult for the average individual who does not have the time or resources to determine the actual facts. Some of the confusion is caused by hucksters who make claims based on poorly-designed studies which should not be used as a basis for decisions about diet and nutrition. Additional confusion occurs because outdated information, which has been reversed by more current evidence, is still being used as a basis for decisions. However, the greatest deterrents in sorting myth from fact are the advertising experts who try to influence the uninformed individual. They use every means possible to confuse the American public by quoting studies their researchers have conducted or by belittling the research of

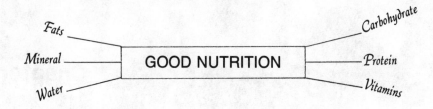

the unbiased nutritionists. These large companies would have you believe that not only is nothing harmful in any of their products but that none of the research is conclusive. The end result is that the average individual does not know what to believe and ultimately does nothing to change his/her diet from the typical American diet. This typical American diet is one of the reasons that Americans have such a high rate of heart disease. There is no nutrient supplement available which supplies all the nutrients essential to life in the amounts in which they are needed. Also, no single class of foods provides what is necessary.

Our goal in this chapter is to help you gain an understanding of nutrition which will enable you to make confident changes in your current eating habits.

UNDERSTANDING THE NUTRIENTS

Nutrients are chemical substances which are obtained from food during digestion. The body requires six basic nutrients: carbohydrates, proteins, fats, vitamins, minerals and water. It is possible to obtain these nutrients from the foods we eat. However, because of present eating habits, many people lack an adequate supply of one or more of these nutrients. Thus, the first step in analyzing the quality of a diet is to gain a meaningful understanding of the role each nutrient plays in helping us achieve optimal health.

Carbohydrates

There are two categories of carbohydrates — sugars and starches. The confusion and concern about carbohydrates in our diet has developed because of the great variability between these two groups. One group is made up of the sugars that are quickly broken down and absorbed by our bodies. These simple carbohydrates include such refined sugars and carbohydrates as white bread, rolls, snack food, candy bars, jellies, and hot fudge sundaes. In addition, a simple carbohydrate found naturally in fruits is more slowly digested and is packed with vitamins, minerals and fibers.

The complex carbohydrates are those identified as the starches which provide a more stable form of energy and have great supplies of other nutrients needed by the body. Generally, complex carbohydrates are found in the natural types of foods: vegetables, cereals, whole grains and beans.

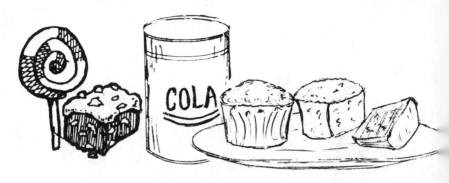

Sugar

It is important to realize the potential problems related to refined carbohydrates. In addition to increased dental problems, dietary sugar causes a rapid elevation of blood sugar, elevation of blood triglycerides, and may stimulate the liver to produce more cholesterol. Because sugar is quickly converted to glucose and rapidly gets into the bloodstream, there may be a short feeling of quick energy. However, the pancreas releases insulin necessary for the utilization of the sugar in such large amounts that the blood sugar level is then driven lower than normal. As a result, you may experience the uncomfortable signs of hypoglycemia: light-headedness, weakness, depression, and even dizziness.

This condition can be even more serious if large amounts of sugar are ingested throughout a lifetime. This places the cells of the pancreas under constant and abnormal stress which leads either to the exhaustion of their ability to synthesize insulin or to the loss of the capacity of tissue cells to absorb the hormone from the bloodstream. The end result can be adult onset diabetes.

Part of the problem with the high intake of refined sugar is the "hidden" sugar in so many foods. Processed foods and beverages account for more than two-thirds of the refined sugar that is consumed. One might be surprised to read the label of many foods and find that sugar has been added. There is also confusion as to whether honey, brown sugar, and molasses are better substitutes for table sugar. For all purposes, honey is still straight sugar; brown sugar is just white sugar with molasses, and raw sugar is no longer available on the market. Blackstrap molasses is the only sugar with anything to offer of nutritional value. It does contain some minerals from the original sugar cane, plus calcium and iron from the processing.

Most people would be wise to observe the following methods of decreasing sugar intake:

1. Drink fewer soft drinks (they average 8 teaspoons per 12 oz.).

2. Eat less baked goods and, when cooking your own, decrease the sugar content.

3. Read food labels and avoid foods containing added sugar.

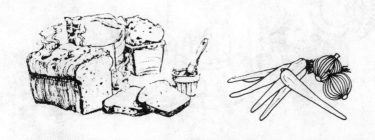

Fiber

Another important component of complex carbohydrates is fiber or roughage. Fiber is the structural part of plants which is neither digested nor absorbed by the body. Dietary fiber is what is left over when food is digested in the human digestive tract. Fiber's most important role is to serve as an intestinal "housecleaner." The added bulk supplied by fiber makes the intestines contract which speeds the food through your digestive system. Since toxic chemicals (including some carcinogens) can be produced by bacteria and enzymes during digestion, this shorter "transit time" helps to move them out faster, perhaps averting cancer of the colon which is associated with low-fiber diets. High-fiber diets also cause the cholesterol to bind with bile acids and then be excreted, which causes a decrease in blood cholesterol level.

Foods that are especially good sources of fiber include bran, oats, wheat, corn, carrots, apples, cabbage, potatoes, turnips, raspberries, blackberries, and seeds.

CARBOHYDRATES (COMPLEX)

Function	Source	Calories per gram	% recommended in diet
Broken down into glucose, which is the major source of energy. Some is stored in liver and muscles in the form of glycogen. Supply fiber	Fruits Vegetables Grains Cereals	4	58% or higher

Note: Limit your intake of refined carbohydrates such as table sugar, sweets, pastries, and soft drinks.

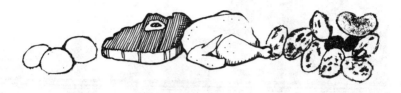

Proteins

Proteins are made up of amino acids needed to build, repair and regulate the function of the body's cells. The body can manufacture some amino acids but not all. Those which must be supplied by the foods we eat each day are known as essential amino acids. Protein foods that contain all the essential amino acids are called complete proteins and are generally foods of animal origin. Those protein foods lacking in certain essential amino acids are referred to as incomplete proteins. However, two or more incomplete proteins can be combined to form a complete protein.

The key factor is providing the body with a variety of foods in a relatively balanced diet. If this occurs the body has the ability to accommodate wide variations in the type and amount of protein it receives and still meet its needs. As a rule, Americans actually consume too much protein.

PROTEINS

Function	Source	Calories per gram	% recommended in diet
Important for growth maintenance and repair of tissue. Also used to form hormones and enzymes; additional source of energy.	*Complete Proteins:* cheese, eggs, milk, chicken, fish, meat. *Incomplete Proteins:* dried peas, beans, legumes, black-eyed peas, soybeans, black beans.	4	10-12%

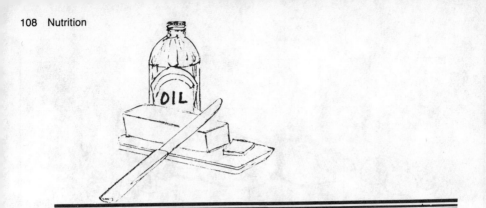

Fats

Some fats are needed by the body because they fulfill several important functions. However, the typical American diet contains over 40% fat as compared to the 20-30% which is currently recommended. In addition, it is important to examine the types of fat included in one's diet.

The basic building blocks of fats are fatty acids. The fatty acids combine with glycerol to form glycerides. When glycerol combines with three fatty acids, it forms triglycerides. The classification of fats is also based on the number of hydrogen atoms combined with the carbon atoms. Saturated fats have the maximum number of hydrogen atoms, and they remain hard at room temperature. Hydrogenation is a process in which a fat or oil is made to react with hydrogen. This results in a more stable fat and is used to convert a liquid polyunsaturated oil to a more solid form. It does not necessarily increase its saturation.

Those fatty acids which the human body requires but cannot produce are called essential fatty acids. They are polyunsaturated fats and can be obtained primarily from vegetable oils. Linoleic acid is the most important essential fatty acid, and it should provide about 2% of the calories in the diet.

Actually, all fats are a mixture of saturated, polyunsaturated and monounsaturated fatty acids. But some foods are higher in one than the other and it is important to know these differences. Dietary rules recommend that only 10% of the calories in one's diet come from saturated fats. So much "invisible" fat is in foods that many people are unaware of just how much they are getting. This is now recognized as a major health problem because every population in the world having a high rate of heart disease eats a diet rich in saturated fat and cholesterol. It has been found that saturated fat is the prime influence on blood cholesterol level — one gram raises it twice as much as an equal amount of polyunsaturated fat.

Another major health hazard is cancer. Studies now link six forms of cancer with dietary fat, including cancer of the breast and colon — two of the top cancer killers in the United States (4).

FATS

Function	Source	Calories per gram	% recommended in diet
Part of the structure of every cell. Stored energy. Supplies essential fatty acids. Provides and carries fat-soluble vitamins A, D, E, K	*Unsaturated:* Safflower oil, Corn oil, Sunflower oil, Soybean oil, Margarines (made with veg. oils). *Saturated:* Solid and hydrogenated shortening, Coconut oil, Cocoa butter, Palm oil, Butter, cheese, Meat, milk. *Monounsaturated:* Olive oil, Peanut oil.	9	20-30% 10% poly-unsaturated 10% mono unsaturated

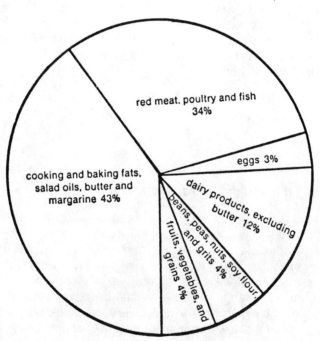

Sources of Fat in the American Diet

"Nutrient Content of the National Food Supply," R. Marston, L. Page. *National Food Review,* pp. 28-33, U.S. Department of Agriculture, December 1978.

Cholesterol

Cholesterol is a waxy, fatty-like material utilized by the body in many chemical processes. Even though cholesterol has no calories as fat does, scientists often refer to it as a fat because it has similar effects on the body. Cholesterol has many important functions in the body: it is a key part of brain tissue, it helps protect nerve fibers, it is necessary for sex hormones as well as other hormones, it helps your body make Vitamin D, and it is necessary for the membranes of all body cells. Actually, cholesterol is such a vital substance that almost every cell in the body manufactures it.

Cholesterol is carried through the blood by a series of molecules called lipoproteins. The low density lipoproteins (LDLs) pick up cholesterol that originates from our diet or is manufactured in the liver and deposits it in the cells for processing. If there is more cholesterol than is needed for daily metabolism, the LDLs may deposit this fatty cargo on the lining of the arteries. These deposits may narrow the arteries in the heart and cause a fatty plaque to build up along the artery. This not only causes the heart to strain in order to pump blood, but may cause a clot which dislodges from an artery and flows through the bloodstream. This clot may eventually lodge in a coronary artery causing reduction of blood flow to the heart muscle and perhaps death from a heart attack. However, high density lipoproteins float around in the bloodstream and pick up the excess cholesterol and carry it back to the liver for excretion from the body. Obviously, our goal is to try to increase our levels of HDL in the blood. Studies show this can be done by:

1. eating a low fat, low cholesterol diet

2. vigorous exercise

3. not smoking

4. avoiding obesity

5. moderate drinking (fewer than 2 drinks a day)

It is important to point out that the effects of consumption of dietary cholesterol do vary from person to person. Some individuals may be lucky enough to maintain a low blood cholesterol level regardless of their diet, but these people are definitely the exception to the rule. Obviously there are many factors that can influence one's blood cholesterol level, and we presently do not completely understand just how a change in this level can be brought about. It does not seem, for instance, that a high dietary intake will depress the body's synthesis of cholesterol to the point that it will cancel out the effect of diet. Some studies now reveal that stress causes an increase in cholesterol production and that a Vitamin C deficiency inhibits the removal of cholesterol from the blood as it passes through the liver.

In regard to an optimal level for blood cholesterol, it seems that below 180 (per 100 ml of blood) an individual's risk of heart disease is low. This risk starts to rise slowly with increasing blood cholesterol levels. Above a level of 250, one's heart attack risk jumps sharply. However, no blood cholesterol level can guarantee to prevent a heart attack. It is not now possible to draw a line between safe and unsafe. We can predict that the chances or odds of suffering a heart attack rise as the cholesterol level rises (4). Although we still have many unanswered questions, most research has shown that a low-fat, low cholesterol diet may be the best way to prevent heart disease. The following agencies have determined that there is enough evidence to strongly advocate this diet for all Americans: U.S. Dept. of Agriculture, Dept. of Health, Education, and Welfare, Senate Select Committee on Nutrition & Human Needs, American Heart Association, American Health Association, National Heart, Lung & Blood Institute, and Center for Science in the Public Interest.

Sources of Cholesterol in the American Diet

Based on: Stamler, J., in *Reprints from Ischaemic Heart Disease*, FADL-Forlag, 1977.

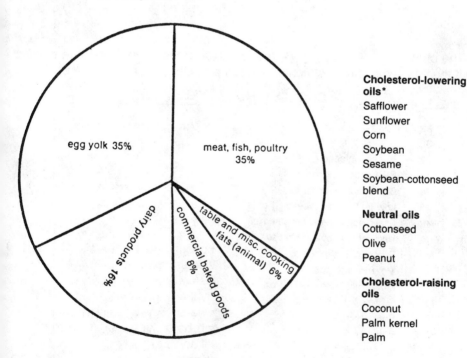

Cholesterol-lowering oils*
Safflower
Sunflower
Corn
Soybean
Sesame
Soybean-cottonseed blend

Neutral oils
Cottonseed
Olive
Peanut

Cholesterol-raising oils
Coconut
Palm kernel
Palm

*In order of polyunsaturated fat content, starting with most polyunsaturated.

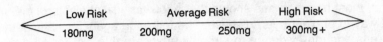

Blood Cholesterol Level

The only foods high in cholesterol are those from animal sources. Therefore, a low cholesterol intake involves **lowering** our consumption of the following: eggs (no more than 3 per week), shrimp, caviar, red meat, all organ and gland meats.

The chart which follows shows the typical sources of cholesterol in our diet and the specific cholesterol count found in a number of common foods.

CHOLESTEROL LEVELS

Mg.	Food	Mg.	Food
35	Butter - 1 T	80	Beef - 3 oz.
22	Butter, whipped - 1 T	63	Chicken - 1/2 breast
24	Bleu cheese - 1 oz.	114	Clams - 1 c.
28	Cheddar cheese - 1 oz.	34	Frankfurter - 1
23	Low fat cottage cheese - 1 c.	83	Lamb - 3 oz.
48	Creamed cottage cheese - 1 c.	372	Liver - 3 oz.
13	Uncreamed cottage cheese - 1 c.	123	Lobster - 1 c.
16	Cream cheese - 1 T	120	Oysters - 1 c.
27	Mozzarella - 1 oz.	76	Pork - 3 oz.
18	Mozzarella, part skim - 1 oz.	192	Shrimp - 1 c.
35	Swiss - 1 1/4 oz. slice	102	Tuna - 1 can
8	Sour cream - 1 T	65	Turkey, light - 3 oz.
252	Egg - whole	86	Turkey, dark - 3 oz.
53	Ice cream - 1 c.	0	Margarine
26	Ice Milk - 1 c.		Milk
34	Milk - 1 c.	79	Evaporated - 1 c.
22	Low-fat milk (2%) 1 c.	105	Condensed - 1 c.
5	Non-fat milk - 1 c.	10	Mayonnaise - 1 T
120	Skim milk - 1 c.	17	Yogurt, non-fat 8 oz.

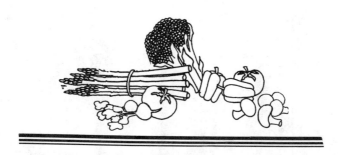

VITAMINS

A vitamin is an organic substance essential for the body to perform its complex chemical reactions. Vitamins cannot be synthesized by the body and are not nutrients in the sense of supplying energy or building tissue, but they aid in the utilization and absorption of the nutrients. Each vitamin performs one or more specific function in the body. Vitamins are divided into two groups on the basis of their solubility. The fat-soluble vitamins A, D, E, and K, are those found in foods associated with fats. They tend to remain stored in the body in moderate quantities. The water soluble vitamins are B and C and are transported in the fluids of the tissues and cells and are not stored in the body in appreciable quantities. The chart which follows describes each vitamin and gives specific information about its function, best sources, and daily requirements.

An important question many people ask is whether the use of a vitamin supplement is recommended. The following reasons have been given to support the need for a supplement:

1. The body's demand for vitamins may increase depending on the stresses and physical activities of the day.

2. One's intake of dietary vitamins may vary — particularly when eating away from home, smoking, and consuming alcoholic beverages.

3. The RDAs cannot serve as an absolute indicator of the adequacy of a given intake for a given individual.

MDR and RDA

As a guide to an adequate intake of the various nutrients, the Minimum Daily Requirement (MDR) and Recommended Dietary Allowance (RDA) have been established. The MDRs were established by the Food and Drug Administration and are average levels, with a small safety margin, required to prevent symptoms of actual deficiency. The RDAs were developed by the Food and Nutrition Board of the National Academy of Sciences and are higher than the MDRs. Actually, a reliable test for determining individual requirements has not yet been devised.

VITAMIN INFORMATION

Vitamin	Food Sources	Deficiency Effect	Function	RDA (Adults)
A	Fish-liver oils, liver, butter, cream, whole milk, whole-milk cheeses, egg yolk, dark-green leafy vegetables, yellow fruits and vegetables.	Night blindness, eye inflammation, dry, rough skin, reduced resistance to infection.	Needed for normal vision. Protects against night blindness. Keeps skin and mucous membranes resistant to infection.	5000 IU
B Complex B₁ (Thiamine)	Pork, liver, organ meats, brewer's yeast, wheat germ, whole-grain cereals and breads, enriched cereals and breads, soybeans, peanuts and other legumes, milk.	Beriberi.	Promotes normal appetite and digestion. Necessary for a healthy nervous system.	1.5 mg.
B₂ (Riboflavin)	Milk, powdered whey, liver, organ meats, meats, eggs, leafy green vegetables, dried yeast, enriched foods.	Cracks at corners of mouth, inflamed, sore lips, inflamed, discolored tongue, dermatitis, anemia.	Helps cells use oxygen. Helps maintain good vision. Needed for good skin.	1.7 mg.
Niacin	Lean meat, fish, poultry, liver, kidney, whole-grain and enriched cereals and breads, green vegetables, peanuts, brewer's yeast.	Pellagra.	Aids metabolism of proteins, carbos, fats.	20 mg.
Pantothenic Acid	Present in most plant and animal tissue, liver, kidney, yeast, eggs, peanuts, whole-grain cereals, beef, tomatoes, broccoli, salmon.	(Rare) Gastrointestinal disturbance, depression, confusion.	Necessary for metabolism of proteins, carbos, fats.	10 mg.
B₆ (Pyridoxine)	Wheat germ, meat, liver, kidney, whole-grain cereals, soybeans, peanuts, corn.	(Rare) Inflamed mouth and tongue, depression, irritability, convulsions.	Maintains normal hemoglobin (carries oxygen to tissues).	2.0 mg.
Biotin	Liver, sweetbreads, yeast, eggs, legumes.	(Extremely rare) Inflamed skin, hair loss, lethargy, loss of appetite.	Coenzyme, functions in metabolism of major nutrients.	0.3 mg.

Adapted from the following sources: 1980 Recommended Daily Dietary Allowances, Food and Nutrition Board, National Academy of Sciences — National Research Council; Runner's World, April 1981.

MINERALS

Minerals are inorganic nutrients which are important in activating numerous reactions that release energy during the breakdown of carbohydrates, proteins, and fats. There are six macrominerals required in larger quantities than the others: sodium, potassium, chloride, calcium, phosphorus, and magnesium. These are needed in the diet in amounts of 100 mg. or more per day. There are 14 others, called trace minerals, which are required in amounts from 100 mg. per day to as little as a few micrograms.

Minerals are supplied by the foods we eat and by the water we drink. The quantities needed are small: the total amount of minerals needed in a day is approximately 200 mg., which could be the size of a pea or a small pill, while those needed in the microgram range could be as tiny as a grain of sand.

The following chart describes each mineral and provides information about its function, sources, and RDA.

MINERAL REQUIREMENTS

MINERALS	WHAT IT DOES	R.D.A.	GOOD SOURCES
CALCIUM	Developing & maintaining strong bones & teeth — normal blood clotting, heartbeat, transmission of nerve impulses, & muscle contraction	800 mg.	milk & milk products green leafy vegetables, almonds
PHOSPHORUS	Utilization of energy, muscle action, & nerve transmission. With calcium, essential for formation of bones, & teeth	800 mg.	meat, poultry, fish, eggs, & whole grain foods
MAGNESIUM	Essential for energy conversions in the body. Helps control muscle contractions.	300 - 350 mg.	dark bread, nuts, green leafy vegetables, dairy products.
POTASSIUM	With sodium it helps regulate the balance and volume of body fluids.	1875 - 5625 mg.	all fruits & vegetables, pecans & walnuts, wheat germ, soybeans, & molasses
SODIUM	Found in blood plasma & other fluids outside cells — helps to maintain normal water balance	1100 - 3300 mg.	meat, fish, poultry, eggs, and milk
CHLORIDE (Mainly in compound form with sodium or potassium)	Regulates correct balance of acid & alkali in blood. Stimulates production of hydrochloric acid in stomach for disgestion	1700 - 5100 mg.	table salt, kelp, ripe olives & rye flour
IRON	Red Blood Cell Formation	18 mg.	eggs, liver, whole grains, dried fruits & legumes

continued

ZINC	Protein synthesis, growth, and development	15 mg.	fish, beef, chicken, whole grains, vegetables, & oysters
IODINE	Functioning of thyroid gland (breathing rate of tissues)	150 mcg.	seafoods
COPPER	Action of enzyme systems & normal functioning of central nervous system — Involved with storage & release of iron to form hemoglobin.	2.0 - 3.0 mg.	organ meats, shellfish nuts, & dried legumes
SELENIUM	Functioning of kidneys, pancreas, and liver.	.05 - 0.2 mg.	organ meats, muscle and seafoods
MANGANESE	Normal tendon & bone structure	2.5 - 5.0 mg.	peas, beans, nuts, fruits, & whole grains

Salt

Salt is an essential mineral nutrient composed of sodium and chloride. We need the electrolyte, sodium, to help maintain a proper fluid balance in our blood and tissues and the acid base balance outside the body cells. However, an excessive intake forces the kidneys to work overtime and contributes to bloating, tissue swelling, and menstrual discomforts. In addition, the relationship of salt to the development of high blood pressure is now well documented. Studies show a worldwide correlation between the quantity of salt ingested and the incidence of hypertension in the population. In those countries where a low amount of salt is consumed, there is a corresponding low incidence of hypertension. (6) While our actual physiological requirement for sodium is only 220 mg. (or about 1/10 of a teaspoon), the average American consumes 10-20 grams (the equivalent of 2-4 teaspoons) of salt per day.

The problem is that we really can't tell how much salt is in the processed foods we eat. However, we do know that salt is needlessly added to many foods by the processors. This is why canned and ready-to-eat foods increase our sodium intake enormously. Therefore, in order to reduce salt intake we suggest:

1. Reduce use of salt in cooking and at the table.

2. Choose foods that have not been processed (fresh fruits and vegetables).

3. Reduce consumption of foods containing visible salt (potato chips, pretzels, salted nuts, corn chips, etc.).

4. Reduce consumption of processed foods (canned vegetables, snack foods, T.V. dinners). (5)

WATER

Although water carries no food value, it is essential for transporting materials and provides a medium within the cell in which the cell's chemical reaction takes place. It is recommended that two to three quarts of water be ingested each day to assist in the digestion of food, excretion, glandular secretion, and formation of blood plasma. Water also helps regulate body temperature (by evaporation through the skin).

It is especially important that persons involved in strenuous exercise programs take care to replace the water lost through perspiration. A good rule to follow would be to drink *at least* one large glass of water before and after exercise. Another suggestion is to make it a habit to stop and drink at every water fountain you pass. Of course, under certain circumstances, this could pose a problem.

THE REVISED BASIC FOUR

Nutritionists have long recognized four basic food groups as being the key to obtaining a well-balanced, nutritious diet. Essentially these food groups can still be used as a guideline for proper eating. However, in view of the information now available concerning the possible dangers of some foods, we need to select carefully those that are low in fat, saturated fat, and cholesterol. Although the groups are not new, our emphasis on which foods are given priority has changed. Instead of selecting any of the foods within a group, we suggest that you give careful consideration to your selection. A fifth group has been added because guidelines are needed for certain common foods usually included in most diets.

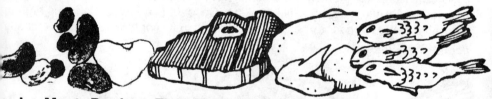

I. Meat, Poultry, Fish, Eggs, Legumes, Nuts

Eat more poultry. The fat of chicken, turkey, and other fowl is more polyunsaturated than the fat of red meats. Chicken and turkey are very lean if the skin is removed, since much of the fat occurs in the skin.

Eat more fish. No fish has a high saturated fat content.

Eat more beans, peas, and lentils. These provide generous amounts of B vitamins and proteins and have almost no fat and no cholesterol (except soybeans).

Eat nuts, seeds, and peanut butter in moderation. Although the fat content is relatively high, the fat of most nuts and seeds is unsaturated.

Eat fewer egg yolks — limit yourself to two or three per week. Replace fatty meat with lean red meat.

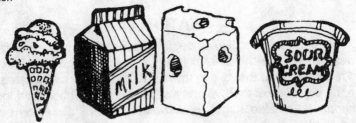

II.   Dairy Products: Milk, Cheese, Ice Cream

Use low-fat or skim milk in cooking and drinking.

Use low-fat cottage cheese.

Use less hard cheese. Use part skim cheeses such as Jarlsberg or Mozzarella.

Try making your own low-fat cream cheese, sour cream, and whipped topping with low-fat ingredients.

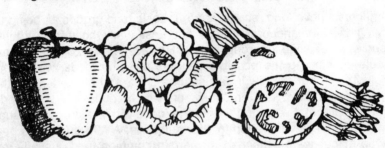

III.   Fruits and Vegetables

All fruits and vegetables are cholesterol-free. Most do not have any fat to speak of unless it is added while cooking. Coconut is an exception. It is high in saturated fat. Avocadoes are also high in fat content but it is mostly monounsaturated.

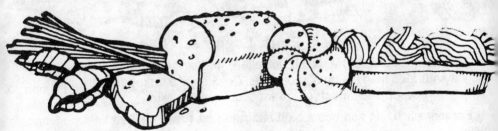

IV.   Bread, Grains, and Cereals

Use grains and cereals made from whole wheat flour or lightly milled.

Use any low-fat flour product.

Use pita breads.

Use breads, cereals, crackers, pasta, tortillas, baked goods and other grain products without added fats, oils, sugars, or egg yolks.

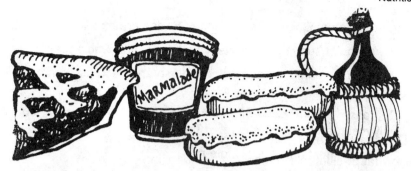

V. The Extras — Fats, Oils, Desserts, and Beverages

Use oils that are highest in polyunsaturated fat: safflower, sunflower, corn oil, etc.

Use diet margarines (half as much fat per tablespoon as regular) and "whipped" margarines.

Avoid all commercial baked goods — make your own low-fat product.

Use cakes and cookies that are low in fat: angel food cake (no fat, no cholesterol), fig bars, and ginger snaps.

Use oil in making pie crusts. Experiment in recipes by cutting the oil, butter, or margarine by a third.

Use vegetable juices, unsweetened fruit juices, and herbal tea.

One final note on the basic food groups. Many people look at the list of foods we are suggesting be eaten less and remark that all the "good" foods are bad for you. No doubt this does appear to be the case, but once you adjust to these new eating habits you will find that other foods will now become "good" — you will acquire a taste for foods that are **less sweet, less salty,** and **less fat.** Also, keep in mind there is a difference in "cutting back" and "cutting out" foods from your diet.

Hopefully, once you are able to distinguish the difference between low quality and high quality food, you will make the choice essential for good health.

RECOMMENDED DIETARY GOALS

In 1977 the U.S. Senate Select Committee on Human Nutrition and Human Needs, chaired by Senator George McGovern, issued a statement on risk factors in the American diet and a proposal for changes in eating habits of Americans. This committee recognized that the changes which had been taking place in the American diet for the past fifty years have not been beneficial to the health of the nation. Never before had a government agency made such specific recommendations on what should be eaten. Although these goals were met with considerable resistance when they were first released (by food industries directly effected by the report — meat, eggs, sugar, etc.), they were soon reinforced by similar dietary guidelines issued by the U.S. Department of Agriculture - Health, Education and Welfare in 1980.

Briefly the "Dietary Goals" for the United States are as follows:

1. Increase consumption of fruits, vegetables, and whole grains.

2. Increase consumption of poultry and fish and decrease consumption of meat.

3. Decrease consumption of foods high in fat, and partially substitute polyunsaturated fat for saturated fat.

4. Substitute nonfat milk for whole milk.

5. Decrease consumption of butter, fat, eggs, and other high cholesterol sources.

6. Decrease consumption of sugar and foods high in sugar content.

7. Decrease consumption of salt and foods high in salt content. (2)

THE LAST WORD

We each control the types and amounts of food we eat. Therefore, we are directly responsible for our body's nutritional state. Through better nutrition we can improve the quailty of all aspects of our lives. Whether at work, in school, in sports or in leisure activities, we will perform only as well as our physical well-being allows. One cannot consistently deprive the body of the essential nutrients it needs, for the effects of a diet deficiency or imbalance are slow and subtle, but inevitable. The choice of good diet and improved nutrition is yours.

REFERENCES

1. Allsen, P.; Harrison, J.; and Vance, B. *Fitness for Life.* Wm. C. Brown Co., Dubuque, Iowa, 1980.

2. Falls, H.; Baylor, A.; and Dishman, R. *Essentials of Fitness.* Saunders College, Philadelphia, 1980.

3. Garrison, Linda and Reed, Ann. *Fitness for Every Body.* Mayfield Publishing Co., Palo Alto, California, 1980.

4. Hausman, Patricia. *Jack Sprat's Legacy.* Richard Marek Publishing Co., New York, 1981.

5. Kapitan, Anne and Wintle, Carol. *Food for the Health of It.* Somerville Public Schools, Sommerville, Massachusetts, 1980.

6. Miller, David K. and Allen, T. Earl. *Fitness: A Lifetime Commitment.* Burgess Publishing Co., Minneapolis, 1982.

Chapter 9

THE BALANCING ACT
■
Weight Control

Knowledge of the basics of nutrition is the first step in learning to eat properly, to attaining (or maintaining) your optimal weight, and to achieving a healthy lifestyle. However, the matter of permanent weight control is not a simple one. This chapter is designed to help you understand the how and why of weight control, and to provide a plan for establishing a program based on your individual needs.

Analyzing Your Body Composition

When it comes to evaluating body composition, scales and height/weight charts can be misleading. All that they really say is whether you have excess weight — body weight that exceeds the normal standards based on height, sex, and frame size. They are not adequate because it is not a person's weight, but what that weight consists of that is important — in other words, how much of your weight is lean mass (bone, muscle, water) and how much is fat. A person could be in the acceptable range according to the height/weight tables but have excessive fat, while a muscular person might be considered overweight yet have very little body fat. For a typical height/weight chart which can be used to determine your correct weight, see page 15.

Our major concern should be that of obesity — excess accumulation of body fat beyond what is considered desirable for a person's sex. The amount of fat can be evaluated by measuring certain body areas using an instrument called "calipers" or by doing a simple "pinch" test. These methods are described in Chapter 2. While most people know they have excess body fat (at least in certain areas), others may be surprised to learn that their body composition is less than ideal — that the weight scale has not told them the whole story. Optimal body fat percentage should not exceed 20% for women or 15% for men.

Unfortunately, a large segment of the American population is obese. Obesity is one of the major health problems in the United States today. The average American gains one pound of weight each year beyond the age of 25, and this gain is in the form of fat! Furthermore, we know there is a high relationship between obesity and increased risk of death from a variety of diseases. Studies show that obesity may not only increase the risk of developing some diseases but may aggravate diseases which are caused by other factors. Specifically, obesity has been linked to the following problems:

1. Every extra pound of fat causes the heart to pump blood through an extra two-thirds of a mile of blood vessels.

2. High blood pressure.

3. Increased level of cholesterol and triglycerides.

4. Many types of bone and joint disorders.

5. Diabetes.

6. Lower back difficulties.

7. Respiratory ailments.

8. Higher incidence of accidents, surgical and pregnancy complications.

There is little doubt that being obese is a threat to the quality and possibly the length of one's life.

The Causes of Obesity

Do you know how obesity develops? What are the major causes of obesity — heredity? Environment? Emotional problems? Lack of activity? Obviously, the answer may vary from individual to individual, and it is likely that more than one cause is involved.

To begin with, we must recognize the role heredity plays. Some individuals are born with more of a *tendency* to become obese. Reasons for this include: (1) an abnormal carbohydrate metabolism; (2) an abnormally efficient fat storing mechanism; (3) physiological traits which are passed on genetically (2); (4) an unusually high number of fat cells.

However, even if there is some genetic tendency to become obese, it is not inevitable. We can control and prevent it!

Our environment may be another factor due to acquired family eating habits or culturally developed attitudes toward weight. Eating patterns which contribute to obesity are typically established early in life. Overeating by young children tends to increase the number of fat cells and contribute to the problem of controlling their weight throughout their lifetime. Since eating habits are established early in life, overfeeding children can be the cause for future weight problems.

Another reason cited for obesity is emotional overeating — the situation in which one turns to food to relieve stress or anxiety. Some individuals use food when they are angry, depressed, bored, frustrated, nervous, or upset for any reason. Anyone caught in this pattern needs to be able to recognize the situation and identify behavior modification methods which can help solve the problem.

Still another factor to consider is that the basal metabolism rate differs among people. The basal metabolism rate is the rate at which the body uses energy to maintain itself while at complete rest, and it declines gradually as one grows older. This rate drops when we sleep, is generally higher in men, and increases as a result of exercise. Therefore, although each of us is different, we do have some means of increasing our basal metabolism rate.

Dr. Jean Mayer, a leading nutritionist, has stated that inactivity is the most important reason for the high incidence of obesity in our modern Western societies. Our sedentary lifestyle has been the major cause of the problem — not overeating. As a matter of fact, it appears that the majority of obese individuals do not eat any more than the non-obese. Clearly, sedentary lifestyles have contributed to the high incidence of obesity. We simply do not have a level of activity that will "burn up" the calories we take in each day. Therefore, the real key to controlling our weight and obesity is being active. We must include a planned exercise program as a part of our daily lives. Keeping our weight at the optimal level is a lifetime activity and for most of us a lifetime of dieting cannot be successful. We must not think in terms of "going on a diet" but in terms of a change in our lifestyles to include increased exercise and improved eating habits.

The Calorie

Since the basic principle of weight control depends on the ratio between caloric intake and caloric expenditure, we need to understand what a calorie is and how many we actually need. The calorie is the common unit of measurement used to express the potential energy of food. Calories are actually by-products of the chemical changes which our bodies produce from the food we eat. We derive calories or energy from fat (9 calories per gram), carbohydrates (4 calories per gram), and protein (4 calories per gram). From these various caloric sources we obtain the energy needed to digest food, conduct our activities, and maintain body heat. The basic energy needs of the body are based on size, age, and type and amount of daily physical activity. If the food we eat provides us with a surplus of calories — more than we can use at the moment — our body has the ability to store these calories for use in the form of fat. One pound of fat is equivalent to 3,500 excess calories.

Determining the precise number of calories required to maintain your ideal weight is not a simple matter; however, you can determine the approximate number of calories needed per day:

1.   Multiply your **ideal** weight by 10 (this determines the number of calories you use at rest — basal metabolic rate or BMR).

2.   Based on your level of activity, add one of the following:
     Sedentary — add 1/3 again of your BMR; Moderately active (90 minutes

of exercise per week) — add 1/2 again your BMR; Very active (Jog or run 5 miles a day) — may double your BMR (11).

Men generally have a higher minimum caloric need than women, because of a greater proportion of musculature, less fat, and larger size. More energy is required to transform food to energy when more muscle tissue is present.

By calculating the number of calories consumed in our diets and the number expended through the BMR and our daily activities, we can determine if caloric balance has been achieved. The following diagram reflects the importance of analyzing caloric intake and expenditure if one is to achieve and maintain the correct weight.

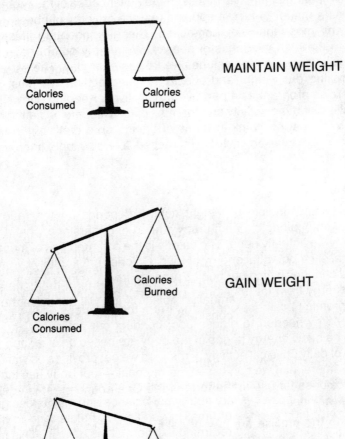

MAINTAIN WEIGHT

Calories Consumed   Calories Burned

GAIN WEIGHT

Calories Burned

Calories Consumed

LOSE WEIGHT

Calories Consumed

Calories Burned

Increasing Calorie Expenditure

When a person has an inactive lifestyle, it is very easy for caloric intake to exceed the energy demands of the body and therefore result in the accumulation of fat deposits. While some may fear that increasing the exercise level will lead to a corresponding increase in appetite, such is not the case. Most studies show that increased activity may stimulate increased food intake but it does not increase above the required energy expenditure. Vigorous, aerobic exercise sustained for an adequate duration will actually cause the body to go beyond the burning of carbohydrates and utilize fat deposits for muscle energy production.

During exercise caloric expenditure can be calculated by measuring the amount of oxygen used in performing the activity. Energy expenditures for different activities vary according to body weight and skill level. Approximations have been prepared from actual measurements and are listed in Appendix J. Generally speaking, exercising with more intensity in a given activity does not increase the caloric expenditure as much as exercising longer and/or covering more distance. (12)

Milkshake Diet   Grapefruit Diet   Beverly Hills Diet   Rice Diet

Fad Diets

Fad diets are extremely popular because everyone is looking for a quick easy way to achieve weight control. However, fad dieting ultimately leads to failure because it usually does not result in a permanent weight loss. The main shortcoming of fad diets is that they do not bring about a change in basic eating habits and lifestyle. Losing weight is not a temporary, short-term problem, so "going on" a diet (and, of course, eventually "going off it") will not solve the problem. To be effective, a diet must be considered from a long-range view of establishing permanent eating habits that will lead not only to weight control but to a healthy life. Therefore, the best strategy for a lifetime of successful weight control is a sound, nutritious diet combined with regular, vigorous exercise.

Actually it is fortunate that so few people can stay on a fad diet. Most quick-reducing diets lack the necessary nutritional balance and may cause great harm if adhered to for long periods of time. In addition, fad diets tend to disturb the body's metabolic balance and returning to "normal" is difficult. This may cause the individual to deposit more fat than usual after going off the diet. Some diets even make the claim that they provide a special metabolic combination of foods which accelerates weight loss. There is no such magic combination just as no one food can help break down fat. Also, remember there is no such thing as a "fattening food" — it is the total number of calories in all foods eaten that determines whether you gain weight. Fat deposits can result from excess calories from any source — carbohydrates, proteins, and alcohol, as well as fats.

Fasting

Some people mistakenly seek semi-starvation or fasting as a means of quick weight loss. The weight loss experienced with fasting and other drastic measures is mainly lean body mass or muscle. Fasting tends to confuse the body and it starts burning up the wrong tissues. Research clearly shows that when fasting only one-third of the weight loss is fatty tissue, while two-thirds is lean body tissue. The reason for this occurrence is that when energy intake is too low, the body maintains the blood glucose level by converting the available amino acids in muscle tissue to glucose.

Another problem arising from extreme caloric deprivation is that the body decreases its metabolic rate. Therefore, calories are burned more slowly and even an extremely small number of calories are sufficient to maintain one's weight. This also triggers the mechanism which causes the body to store fat more efficiently, thus a decrease in lean muscle tissue and an increase in fat storage, to say nothing of the potential health problems which an individual can suffer through a prolonged or consistent program of fasting. Fasting is certainly not recommended as an approach to effective and safe weight loss.

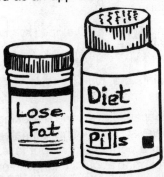

Diet Aids (Pills, Candy, Gum, etc.)

The basic problem with all diet aids is similar to that of fad diets — they do not meet the nutritional needs of the individual and they do not bring about a change in the basic eating habits of the individual. The goals of such aids are to curb the appetite, numb the taste buds, or provide a feeling of fullness. Most pills contain a drug called phenylpropanolamine (PPA) which your body can build a tolerance to and which lead to psychological dependence. Some pills have caffeine to relieve feelings of fatigue or diuretics which cause only water weight loss. The chewing gum or candy-type diet aids depend on benzocaine, a mild topical anesthetic, to numb your taste buds.

Just because a diet aid is sold over the counter doesn't mean it is completely safe. Certain individuals may be susceptible to a particular chemical, may unintentionally overdose on a drug which is found in other medications being taken, and some may develop other side effects. Obviously, however, the major drawback is that such an approach does not contribute to a permanent weight loss.

GUIDELINES FOR PERMANENT WEIGHT CONTROL

As stated previously, permanent weight control is most effectively achieved through a program of sound nutrition and regular exercise. The goal is to develop a habit of good eating and activity that is a daily part of our lives. Basic guidelines which should be considered in establishing a program for permanent weight control are as follows:

1. The program should be based on an analysis of current eating and exercise habits so that specific modifications in your lifestyle can be adapted which will be maintained throughout life.

2. For weight loss the total calorie intake should be less than the total calories "burned" (negative caloric balance).

3. The diet should contain the percentage of required nutrients established for an optimal diet (See Chapter 5).

4. Weight loss will generally be more lasting if it is gradual. A safe recommendation is to lose no more than one to two pounds per week unless under a doctor's supervision.

5. A regular exercise program should be developed to maximize the calorie expenditure and the loss of fat tissue (1).

6. Try to select foods providing the highest food value for the fewest calories; i.e., high in vitamins and minerals but low in fat. Make the most of the calories included in your diet.

7. Avoid trying fad diets or "quick" weight loss programs that may be worthless and dangerous.

8. Attempt to balance your caloric intake throughout the day rather than in one or two heavy meals.

9. Remember that your weight loss may not follow a steady rate. Your body may make changes and adjustments that could lead you to believe your diet is not working. So don't be discouraged.

10. Caloric intake of fewer than 1500 calories per day for men and 1200 calories per day for women is not recommended as safe over long periods of time.

Analyzing Your Calorie Needs

A basic approach to improving your diet and establishing a method of weight control is to analyze your caloric intake and expenditure. It is important to remove all guesswork from the process, and base your decisions on accurate knowledge of your specific needs.

Most people have a very inaccurate concept of their caloric intake. Even those who appear to be calorie conscious need to keep specific records to maintain accuracy. Therefore, the first recommendation is to collect information about your daily food intake. Lab 7 will assist you in gathering the needed information and help you recognize the patterns, problems, and possible solutions to improving your diet plan. Although time-consuming, this project reveals important information which is needed for assistance in establishing a long-term approach to permanent weight control.

The next step is to analyze your caloric expenditure. Lab 8 in the Appendix will enable you to calculate your current calorie needs as well as identify future exercise programs to increase this expenditure.

As stated at the beginning of this chapter, the key to weight control is balancing caloric intake and expenditure. By knowing your caloric needs, by carefully analyzing your daily food intake, and by determining your potential caloric expenditure, you can achieve your goal more quickly without the risk of jeopardizing your overall health. It may not be easy and it may require some sacrifices on your part, but if you really make the commitment the results are sure.

REFERENCES

1. Allsen, P.; Harrison, J.; and Vance, B. *Fitness for Life.* Wm. C. Brown Co., Dubuque, Iowa, 1980.

2. Dusek, Dorothy. *Thin and Fit: Your Personal Lifestyle.* Wadsworth Publishing Co., Belmont, California, 1982.

3. Fisher, A. Garth and Conlee, Robert K. *The Complete Book of Physical Fitness.* Brigham Young University Press, Utah, 1979.

4. Garrison, L.; Leslie, P.; and Blackmore, D. *Fitness and Figure Control.* Mayfield Publishing Co., Palo Alto, California, 1981.

5. Garrison, Linda and Reed, Ann. *Fitness for Every Body.* Mayfield Publishing Co., Palo Alto, California 1980.

6. Getchell, Bud. *Being Fit — A Personal Guide.* John Wiley & Sons, New York, 1982.

7. Getchell, Bud. *Physical Fitness: A Way of Life.* John Wiley & Sons, New York, 1976.

8. Hockey, Robert V. *Physical Fitness — The Pathway to Healthful Living.* C. V. Mosby Co., St. Louis, 1981.

9. Lindsey, R.; Jones, B.; and Whitley, A. *Body Mechanics.* Wm. C. Brown Co., Dubuque, Iowa, 1979.

10. Miller, David and Allen, Earl. *Fitness: A Lifetime Commitment.* Burgess Publishing Co., Minneapolis, 1982.

11. Sharkey, Brian. *Physiology of Fitness.* Human Kinetics Pub., Champaign, Illinois, 1979.

12. U.S. Dept. of Health and Human Services. *Exercise and Your Heart.* U.S. Government Printing Office, Washington, 1981.

Chapter 10

COMPLETING THE PICTURE
■
A Plan for Stress Reduction

Realization

The first step in combating stress is realizing there are countless circumstances in every person's daily life which can produce tension or stress. It also helps to understand that these circumstances, with their resulting stress, may cause a mental and physical drain in humans somewhat like a car battery that is not recharging properly. Of course, if the situation is not corrected there will be an eventual breakdown.

Recognition

The second step in the process of stress reduction is to develop the ability to recognize things in *your* life which seem to be causing the most problems, and also being able to recognize symptoms of stress in yourself and others. Some of the tell-tale signs are as follows: (1) curling toes when sitting; (2) drumming fingers on table or desk top; (3) excessive twisting or clasping of hands and fingers; (4) frequent headaches; (5) always feeling tired; (6) difficulty in sleeping; (7) constipation; (8) frequent outbursts of anger; (9) a constant backache or stiff neck. Dr. Kenneth Cooper suggests checking the heart rate early in the morning and then later in the day. A normal increase would be about 10 beats; however, if the rate is increasing 20-30 beats, there are problems.

Resolving the Problem

The following tips and ideas are designed to suggest ways to cope with stress-filled encounters.

- Tune up your fitness level; exercise and work out to produce fatigue and reduce stress.
- Burn up stress by participating in aerobic exercise programs.
- Learn a new type of leisure activity.
- Take a long walk (beach, park, shopping mall); enjoy nature as much as possible.
- Listen to your favorite music.
- Whistle, hum, sing or yell.
- Take a warm bath or a long shower.
- Be with a loving pet.
- Cook something splendid.
- Take yoga lessons.
- Relive great moments in your life.
- Join a crafts class.
- Visit the zoo or a local place of enjoyment and attraction.

Relaxation Techniques

1. Perform stretching exercises slowly with great concentration upon your muscle tension, relaxation, and sense of breathing.

2. Lying on your back, perform a contraction for 6-8 seconds and then allow a sudden release of the tension in various body parts; repeat several times for each body part. Begin in legs and thighs; work the hips, stomach and spine press; go to each leg and arm separately, then move both legs and arms together, then perform a total body stretch, controlling the tension and then performing the gradual releasing of each tension.

3. Lying on your back (bent knee position) perform shoulder lifts, one arm alternately, then both; then release the contraction with a sudden letting go of the held energy.

4. Lying on your back (bent knee position), concentrate on breathing; take a deep inhalation, pushing out the abdominal wall, then deliberately blow air from your mouth while pulling the stomach in tight and pressing the spine against the floor. Perform 4 times and then gradually relax and concentrate on letting go of your tension.

5. Choose a comfortable position as you lie on the floor; preferably bend

your knees up and prop them (as a lean) against one another so that they rest in a relaxed state; hug your arms around yourself and place your hands on the shoulder region; close your eyes and concentrate on an idea or a place that is wonderful for you to remember or think about (i.e., take yourself on a walk through the woods, at the beach, or at a park; pretend to be gazing at a cloud formation; take a ride in your mind's eye.) Caution: Each time your mind is distracted or when it loses its dream-like activity, focus your thoughts on your breathing and count your breaths until you wish to return to what you were thinking about. Enjoy the most of your relaxation moments!

Note: Many of these relaxation activities may be practiced at home or in a classroom while listening to soothing and pleasant background music to enhance your technical practice.

Perform stretching exercises with slow deliberation when concluding a relaxation technique work out.

Recheck Your Health Status

1.   Obtain regular medical checkups.

2.   Have regular dental checkups.

3.   Consider your personal habits of hygiene and health.

4.   Eat sensibly (vary the Basic Nutritional Foods).

5.   Limit the intake of sugars, salts and fats.

6.   Control your weight.

7.   Drink plenty of water daily.

Retire From Stress

1.   Learn to relax with proper methods and techniques.

2.   Talk and communicate with friends and colleagues.

3.   Realize what bugs you.

4.   Plan time for you.

5.   Attempt to resolve bad situations without emotional hangups.

Rest

1.   Establish priorities in order to help you plan adequate rest and sleep needs.

2.   Prevent injuries with proper amounts of rest and sleep.

3.   Prevent mental and physical exhaustion by practicing adequate rest and sound habits.

Return and Remake

We all know how important it is to keep a handle on ourselves and our emotions. Similarly we need to keep a check on our stress-based lives by having a safety exhaust valve that will enable us to ventilate and maintain a safe level. It is important that we learn to vent our pent up tensions and emotions, to recognize causes, and to create practical methods for correcting such disorders in ourselves. Let's find a time, a place and a way . . . to remake ourselves into beings we wish to be and return to a wellness order of life we wish to live.

Rejoice

Having an opportunity to create a fresh new situation, and/or approach to many critical and stressful circumstances in our lives, is a positive action desired by all humans. Let us recognize our shortcomings and learn to adjust and cope to life's stressful ways. Let us be aware that relaxation and rest can be important integrals in rounding out our life style.

The materials presented in this chapter can assist you in developing a completeness to your total fitness. Help yourself to hold on to your life.

REFERENCES

1. Curtis, J. and Detert, R. *How to Relax.* Mayfield Publishing Co., Palo Alto, California, 1981.

2. Garrison, Linda; Leslie, Phyllis; and Blackmore, Deborah L. *Fitness and Figure Control: The Creation of You (2nd ed.).* Mayfield Publishing Co., Palo Alto, California, 1981.

3. Gray, Miriam. *Physical Education Demonstration.* A. S. Barnes, New York, 1947.

4. Loren, Teri. *The Dancer's Companion: The Indispensable Guide to Getting the Most Out of Dance Classes.* Dial, New York, 1978.

5. Peale, Norman Vincent. *Stay Alive All Your Life.* Fawcett, Greenwich, Connecticut, 1957.

6. Penrod, James and Plastino, Janice Gudde. *The Dancer Prepares: Modern Dance for Beginners.* Mayfield Publishing Co., Palo Alto, California, 1980.

Chapter 11

FILLING THE GAPS
■
Questions and Answers

Is a physical examination necessary before I begin my exercise program?

Although it is advisable to evaluate your physical condition, in most cases people below the age of 35 do not need a physical examination before exercising. If you plan a gradual, sensible exercise program, there are minimal health risks. However, individuals with the following symptoms should seek medical advice: (1) heart trouble, heart murmur; (2) frequent pains or pressure — in left or midchest area, left neck; (3) often feel faint or have spells of severe dizziness; (4) experience extreme breathlessness after mild exertion; (5) blood pressure too high and is not under control; (6) bone or joint problems such as arthritis; (7) over age 35-40 and not accustomed to vigorous exercise; (8) a family history of premature coronary artery disease.

How will I know if I have exceeded the safe limits for exercise?

There are several warning signs which indicate you are over-exercising and should reduce the intensity of the workout: excessive heart rate, labored breathing, pale skin, flushness, and a prolonged heart recovery time after exercising.

Any of the following signs indicate that exercise should be stopped immediately because the participant may be in danger: difficulty in breathing (not just deep breathing); loss of coordination; dizziness; tightness in the chest.

If the participant exhibits any of these danger signs, he/she should seek medical advice before continuing with the exercise program.

Are there any risks to jogging?

Although jogging is an excellent aerobic exercise, it certainly is not appropriate for everyone. The most common risks are injuries to the muscles and joints. These injuries tend to occur more frequently when you exercise too intensely, if you have been inactive for a period of time, or if you are excessively overweight. Jogging in inadequate shoes or on hard surfaces can also cause problems. However, by following the guidelines suggested in Chapter 4, most of these injuries can be prevented.

How does exercise contribute to weight control?

Exercise can play an important role in your effort to regulate weight. Not only does the exercise burn calories but it also helps maintain muscle tone and shape. An added benefit can be improvement in the body's ability to burn fat. Vigorous exercise over a period of time enables the body to more efficiently use its stores of fat as muscle fuel. The body's ability to burn fat does improve with exercise.

Does it really matter which exercises I choose to do?

All exercises are not the same. Not only do some exercises burn more calories per minute, but exercises provide benefits which are specific to the type of exercise. For instance, stretching exercises will only contribute to a gain in flexibility — not to strength or endurance. The exercises requiring continuous activity and involving large muscle groups will provide the greatest caloric expenditure. Therefore, you must select exercises which meet your needs — whether it is for a specific fitness component or for weight control.

Can I spot reduce?

It is now very clear that one *cannot* spot reduce. Exercising the muscles in a particular area will not cause the fat around that muscle to be broken down for energy. During vigorous exercise the muscles call upon fat storage deposits throughout the body for fuel. Heredity determines our particular distribution of fat deposits. That is the reason each of us gains weight in different areas. The best way to lose fat is to participate in vigorous activity that can be sustained for long periods of time.

What causes muscle soreness?

Most muscle soreness occurs between 24-48 hours after the exercise. Although the specific cause is not known, it appears to be due to small tears in the muscle or the connective tissue around the muscle. Previous theories linked the soreness to a buildup of lactic acid in the muscle during sustained activity. In any case, you can help prevent the pain and stiffness by proper warm-up and cool-down, by gradually getting into your exercise program, by progressing slowly, and by avoiding ballistic or bouncing-type stretching exercises.

What can I do for shin splints?

Shin splints refer to the generalized pain in front of the lower leg and are particularly common in runners. The basic cause of shin splints is a muscle imbalance when the calf muscles are stronger than the shin muscles. The recommended treatment is to strengthen the weaker shin muscles and to stretch the stronger calf muscles. Running up stairs will strengthen the shins and the calves can be stretched by doing wall push-ups (see Chapter 4) or using an inclined plane. Other factors to consider are wearing the correct shoes, running on a softer surface, and your running style — try to run softly and smoothly, hitting with the heel just slightly ahead of the rest of the foot.

What causes the "stitch in the side"?

A "stitch" or sudden, sharp pain in the side or upper part of the abdomen, is a form of muscle cramp. Physicians now believe that a cramp occurs in the diaphragm muscle due to the blood supply being cut off by the pressure from the lungs above and the abdomen below during exercise. The muscle goes into a spasm when it is unable to get enough oxygen. You can help prevent a "stitch" by strengthening your diaphragm and abdominal muscles. To relieve the pain, slow down and push your fingers deep into the site of the pain, just below the last rib on the upper right part of the abdomen. Now bend forward and exhale, puckering your lips. When the pain disappears you can continue running.

What special precautions should I take on a hot, humid day?

The body does need time to adapt to hot weather conditions. Even though you might be physically fit, you can only increase your tolerance to heat by exercising regularly in hot weather. Therefore the following steps are recommended:

1. Plan your workouts for the coolest part of the day, such as early morning or early evening after the sun has gone down.

2. Cut back on your workouts — duration and intensity — until you become adapted to the heat.

3. Drink plenty of fluids — especially water.

4. Dress in light-weight, loose-fitting clothing.

5. Never wear rubberized clothing, plastic suits, sweatshirts or sweat pants.

What are the symptoms of heat exhaustion and heat stroke?

The usual symptoms of heat exhaustion include abnormally low body temperature, dizziness, headache, nausea and, sometimes, mental confusion. Symptoms of heat stroke include dizziness, headache, thirst, nausea, muscle cramps, and three important symptoms: sweating stops, a dangerously high

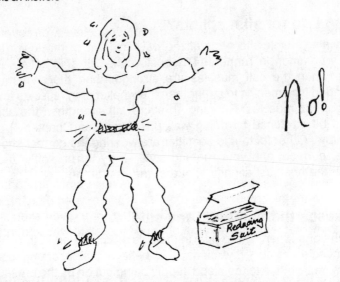

body temperature develops, and unconsciousness frequently occurs. This condition can be very serious. Since excessive body temperature can cause brain damage and even death, medical attention is critical for heat stroke.

What are the dangers of rubberized or plastic clothing?

Many people in their eagerness to lose weight mistake water loss caused by excessive sweating with fat loss. The excessive dehydration caused by wearing rubberized or plastic clothing can be extremely dangerous and does not contribute to a permanent weight loss. The wearing of such clothing causes the body temperature to rise to a potentially dangerous level because the sweat cannot evaporate and evaporation is the body's cooling mechanism. As the temperature continues to rise, sweating increases, leading to excessive water loss.

Should I take salt tablets?

Contrary to what many people have thought, it is not necessary to increase your intake of salt when exercising during hot weather. Not only do we get enough salt in our normal diets, but the body learns to conserve salt so we are not losing as much as previously believed. Studies now show that sweat is mostly water.

How should I dress on extremely cold days?

It is important to dress appropriately when exercising outside on cold days. Generally the following rules should be observed:

1. Wear one layer less of clothing than you would if you were outside but not exercising.

2. Wear several layers of light clothing rather than one heavy layer.

3. Protect your hands by wearing old mittens, gloves, or cotton socks.
4. Wear a head covering. Up to 40% of your body's heat is lost through the neck and head.

It is also suggested that a brief warm-up before going outside is beneficial.

How does smoking affect my fitness level?

Studies definitely show that smokers cannot achieve as high a level of physical fitness as they could if they didn't smoke. Because smoking contributes to a constriction of the blood vessels and a loss in the oxygen-carrying capacity by the blood, the heart rate response will be higher for a given exercise intensity. Individuals who set a goal to achieve optimal fitness but who continue to smoke will automatically fail to reach that goal.

Does missing a few sessions cause me to lose my fitness?

One does not lose all the gains of an exercise program by missing a few days. However, when you begin exercising again you should start at a lower level. Depending on the number of days you missed and how you feel while exercising, it is suggested you begin at half to two-thirds your usual exercise level. Once you have missed the days, don't worry avout them — just get back on schedule and work toward achieving your goal.

Should I join a health spa?

Before making what could be an expensive membership commitment to a health spa or sport club, you should consider the following factors:

1. Numerous abuses have been reported. Deceptive advertising, high pressure sales tactics, misrepresentation in sales presentations, and restrictive and unfair contract cancellation policies, are but a few.
2. Membership is a long-term commitment and to get your money's worth you have to work out regularly at least two to three times a week.
3. If the site is located more than 20 minutes from your home, don't join.
4. Drop in during the hours you would probably be attending to see if overcrowding will be a problem.
5. Check to be sure the equipment is adequate and the type you need, i.e., weights, exercise bicycles, treadmill.
6. Ask about the instructors and check their credentials and qualifications.
7. Examine the written contract carefully before signing it.
8. Make certain similar facilities are not already available at a lower cost or free at a nearby school, college, YWCA or YMCA.

Should I drink one of the special exercise drinks — Gatorade, ERG, Quick Kick, etc.

You should first understand that sweat is 99.1% water and therefore the body is not losing a significant quantity of the electrolytes (sodium, potassium, magnesium, calcium, and phosphate) which are contained in these drinks. During heavy sweating you actually lose so much water that the remaining electrolytes are more concentrated. It is also important to understand that the replacement of lost fluid is slowed significantly when the ingested fluid contains sugar (whether in the form of glucose, fructose, or sucrose). Therefore, if you do drink commercial preparations such as Gatorade, Instant Replay, etc., they should be diluted to speed their absorption.

What is the best way to breathe when I jog?

The main way is to breathe normally and respond naturally to the increased demands on the body. For maximum ventilation breathe in and out through both mouth and nose. In addition, it will help to relax and feel more comfortable if you periodically and forcibly exhale through the mouth.

Is a protein meal the best source of energy before a workout or athletic event?

No, actually protein digestion is more complex and takes longer than carbohydrate digestion. Therefore, the best meal would be one with a high level of complex carbohydrates. These are broken down slowly and provide the body with energy for a longer period of time. In addition, carbohydrates are stored in the liver and muscles in the form of glycogen which is then readily available for conversion into glucose when extra energy is needed (3).

Does jogging cause problems for women by displacing the uterus or stretching the ligaments in the breasts (causing them to droop)?

There is no evidence to support these fears. Actually, most doctors encourage women to exercise. Women in top physical condition generally have less menstrual discomfort, fewer backaches, fewer colds, less digestive disorders, and less fatigue than women who do not exercise. Women who exercise report greater firmness of the breasts due to loss of body fat and improved tone of the pectoral muscles. Displacement of the uterus is extremely unlikely since it has one of the best shock-absorbing systems in the human body (1).

Is running during pregnancy unsafe?

Most physicians indicate that if women were exercising before pregnancy, there is no reason they cannot continue during pregnancy. Of course, it is advisable to consult with your doctor to determine the exact exercise program for you. It may be necessary to make certain adjustments in your program from time to time.

What differences in the results of training will there be between men and women?

The following physiological differences will affect the training potential of women: (1) smaller heart; (2) slightly lower hemoglobin level; (3) less total muscle mass than men. The effect of the first two differences is a lower potential maximum oxygen uptake because less oxygen will be available to the cells during exercise. The effect of the third difference is less total body strength for women compared to men. In spite of these differences, men and women can participate in the same types of training programs and both can realize improvement in their level of physical fitness.

How can I score excellent on one physical fitness test and only fair on another?

Each fitness component — cardiovascular endurance, flexibility, strength, and muscular endurance — is separate and distinct. There is some interrelationship but achieving a high level in one does not mean you will score high in another. The principle of specificity of training is important to remember; improvement in fitness is specific to the type of training undertaken.

Why are "fast foods" not recommended?

There are three primary problems associated with eating too much "fast foods": salt, fat, and calories. These foods also contain too much sugar and too little fiber and vitamins. Not only are these foods high in calories, but approximately 50% of the calories comes from fat.

Are there any dangers in a vegetarian diet?

If one is a strict vegetarian and avoids all milk products as well as meat, there are potential problems. Unless care is taken, protein intake may be insufficient, a calcium deficiency may result, and vitamin B_{12} intake may be inadequate. On the other side of the picture, vegetarians generally have a diet lower in calories, higher in fiber, and lower in fats.

Will drinking alcoholic beverages affect my exercise and fitness?

In addition to the serious health hazards associated with alcohol consumption (liver and kidney problems), the following effects on exercise and fitness have been identified:

1. Reduction in the body's ability to utilize oxygen for at least 48 hours after consumption.

2. Intake of empty calories — 7 calories per gram with no vitamins and minerals.

3. Potential increase in weight due to the additional calories in the diet.

4.   Increase in the serum triglyceride level.

Those serious about improving their health and fitness should carefully consider these effects.

Which type of exercise will help me burn up the most calories?

The basic rule is that the fuel you burn is governed by the amount of weight you move and the distance you move it. Therefore, the same exercises which contribute to cardiovascular fitness are those which burn the most calories. Select activities which involve total body activity, which are rhythmical, and which can be maintained for a longer time. Aerobic dancing is great!

Can exercise help relieve my menstrual cramps?

Exercise can be one of the best remedies to relieve cramps because it helps improve blood circulation in the uterus. It is also believed that exercise produces release of endorphins, natural opiate-like substances that are produced in the brain and relieve pain just as narcotics do.

REFERENCES

1.   Allsen, P.; Harrison, J.; and Vance, B. *Fitness for Life.* Wm. C. Co., Dubuque, Iowa, 1980.

2.   Darden, Ellington. *Especially for Women.* Leisure Press, West Point, New York, 1977.

3.   Garrison, L.; Leslie, P.; and Blackmore, D. *Fitness and Figure Control.* Mayfield Publishing Co., Palo Alto, California, 1981.

4.   Getchell, Bud. *Being Fit — A Personal Guide.* John Wiley & Sons, New York, 1982.

5.   Golding, Lawrence; Myers, C.; and Sinning, W. *The Y's Way to Physical Fitness.* National Board of YMCA, Chicago, 1982.

6.   Mirkin, Gabe and Hoffman, Marshall. *The Sportsmedicine Book.* Little, Brown & Co., Boston, 1978.

7.   Miller, David and Allen, T. Earl. *Fitness: A Lifetime Commitment.* Burgess Publishing Co., Minneapolis, 1982.

8.   Sharkey, Brian. *Physiology of Fitness.* Human Kinetics Pub. Champaign, Illinois, 1979.

9.   U.S. Dept. of Health and Human Services. *Exercise and Your Heart.* U.S. Government Printing Office, Washington, 1981.

APPENDICES

APPENDIX A. ANALYSIS OF BODY FAT

Described below are the techniques used in obtaining skin fold measurements and diagrams of the specific location of the measurements. By taking the sum of measurements for various sites one can predict the percent of body fat. Individual values at the sites may be used to note changes in body composition that occur.

Directions for taking measurement:

1. All measurements should be taken from the right side of the body.

2. Measurements should be taken prior to exercise since sweating and increased blood flow make measurement more difficult.

3. Three measurements of each area should be taken to assure accuracy.

4. The calipers must be placed next to the thumb and index finger and allowed to close completely before the measurement is recorded.

Location of measurements:

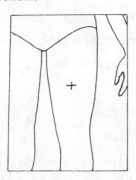

Thigh

A vertical fold midway between the groin line and the patella.

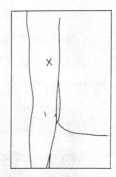

Tricep

A vertical fold midway between the shoulder and elbow joints.

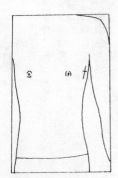

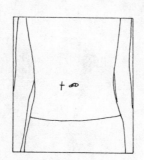

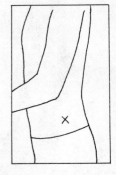

Axilla

A vertical fold on the side at nipple level.

Abdominal

A vertical fold approximately one inch to the right of the navel.

Hip (Ilium)

A diagonal fold just above the crest of the hip bone.

BODY COMPOSITION RATING SCALE
Skinfolds
Norms — Males 35 Years and Younger

Rating	Percent Fat	Chest mm	Abdomen mm	Ilium mm	Axilla mm
Very Lean	6	3	4	4	4
Lean	9	7	8	6	8
Leaner Than Ave.	14	12	16	11	13
Average	18	15	21	16	17
Fatter Than Ave.	22	18	27	20	21
Fat	25	22	34	26	25
Very Fat	30	28	44	33	33

Norms — Males 36-45 Years Old

Rating	Percent Fat	Chest mm	Abdomen mm	Ilium mm	Axilla mm
Very Lean	8	4	6	4	4
Lean	10	8	10	8	10
Leaner Than Ave.	15	13	17	13	15
Average	19	16	22	17	19
Fatter Than Ave.	23	19	28	22	23
Fat	27	24	35	28	28
Very Fat	32	30	45	37	35

Norms — Males 46 Years and Older

Rating	Percent Fat	Chest mm	Abdomen mm	Ilium mm	Axilla mm
Very Lean	9	5	6	6	6
Lean	11	8	11	9	11
Leaner Than Ave.	16	14	18	15	17
Average	21	17	23	19	21
Fatter Than Ave.	24	20	29	23	24
Fat	29	24	36	30	30
Very Fat	34	31	46	39	36

Source: Y's Way To Physical Fitness

BODY COMPOSITION RATING SCALE

Norms — Females 35 Years and Younger

Rating	Percent Fat	Tricep mm	Abdomen mm	Ilium mm
Very Lean	9	5	5	4
Lean	14	7	8	7
Leaner Than Ave.	18	12	14	13
Average	22	15	19	16
Fatter Than Ave.	24	19	25	20
Fat	28	25	33	29
Very Fat	35	30	40	35

Norms — Females 36-45 Years

Rating	Percent Fat	Tricep mm	Abdomen mm	Ilium mm
Very Lean	10	6	6	5
Lean	16	9	8	8
Leaner Than Ave.	20	13	14	14
Average	23	17	19	18
Fatter Than Ave.	26	21	25	21
Fat	31	26	33	29
Very Fat	37	32	40	37

Norms — Females 46 Years and Older

Rating	Percent Fat	Tricep mm	Abdomen mm	Ilium mm
Very Lean	11	8	8	7
Lean	18	10	10	9
Leaner Than Ave.	21	15	15	16
Average	25	18	20	18
Fatter Than Ave.	30	23	26	22
Fat	34	27	35	32
Very Fat	41	34	43	39

Source: Y's Way To Physical Fitness

PERCENT FAT ESTIMATES FOR MEN

Sum of Four Skinfolds

Chest, Ilium, Abdomen, Axilla

Sum of 4 Skinfolds	Age To Last Year								
	18 to 22	23 to 27	28 to 32	33 to 37	38 to 42	43 to 47	48 to 52	53 to 57	58 and older
8-12	1.9	2.5	3.2	3.8	4.4	5.0	5.7	6.3	6.9
13-17	3.3	3.9	4.5	5.1	5.7	6.4	7.0	7.6	8.2
18-22	4.5	5.2	5.8	6.4	7.0	7.7	8.3	8.9	9.5
23-27	5.8	6.4	7.1	7.7	8.3	8.9	9.5	10.2	10.8
28-32	7.1	7.7	8.3	8.9	9.5	10.2	10.8	11.4	12.0
33-37	8.3	8.9	9.5	10.1	10.8	11.4	12.0	12.6	13.2
38-42	9.5	10.1	10.7	11.3	11.9	12.6	13.2	13.8	14.4
43-47	10.6	11.3	11.9	12.5	13.1	13.7	14.4	15.0	15.6
48-52	11.8	12.4	13.0	13.6	14.2	14.9	15.5	16.1	16.7
53-57	12.9	13.5	14.1	14.7	15.4	16.0	16.6	17.2	17.9
58-62	14.0	14.6	15.2	15.8	16.4	17.1	17.7	18.3	18.9
63-67	15.0	15.6	16.3	16.9	17.5	18.1	18.8	19.4	20.0
68-72	16.1	16.7	17.3	17.9	18.5	19.2	19.8	20.4	21.0
73-77	17.1	17.7	18.3	18.9	19.5	20.2	20.8	21.4	22.0
78-82	18.0	18.7	19.3	19.9	20.5	21.0	21.8	22.4	23.0
83-87	19.0	19.6	20.2	20.8	21.5	22.1	22.7	23.3	24.0
88-92	19.9	20.5	21.2	21.8	22.4	23.0	23.6	24.3	24.9
93-97	20.8	21.4	22.1	22.7	23.3	23.9	24.5	25.2	25.8
98-102	21.7	22.3	22.9	23.5	24.2	24.8	25.4	26.0	26.7
103-107	22.5	23.2	23.8	24.4	25.0	25.6	26.3	26.9	27.5
108-112	23.4	24.0	24.6	25.2	25.8	26.5	27.1	27.7	28.3
113-117	24.1	24.8	25.4	26.0	26.6	27.3	27.9	28.5	29.1
118-122	24.9	25.5	26.2	26.8	27.4	28.0	28.6	29.3	29.9
123-127	25.7	26.3	26.9	27.5	28.1	28.8	29.4	30.0	30.6
128-132	26.4	27.0	27.6	28.2	28.8	29.5	30.1	30.7	31.3
133-137	27.1	27.7	28.3	28.9	29.5	30.2	30.8	31.4	32.0
138-142	27.7	28.3	29.0	29.6	30.2	30.8	31.4	32.1	32.7
143-147	28.3	29.0	29.6	30.2	30.8	31.5	32.1	32.7	33.3
148-152	29.0	29.6	30.2	30.8	31.4	32.1	32.7	33.3	33.9
153-157	29.5	30.2	30.8	31.4	32.0	32.7	33.3	33.9	34.5
158-162	30.1	30.7	31.3	31.9	32.6	33.2	33.8	34.4	35.1
163-167	30.6	31.2	31.9	32.5	33.1	33.7	34.3	35.0	35.6
168-172	31.1	31.7	32.4	33.0	33.6	34.2	34.8	35.5	36.1
173-177	31.6	32.2	32.8	33.5	34.1	34.7	35.3	35.9	36.6
178-182	32.0	32.7	33.3	33.9	34.5	35.2	35.8	36.4	37.0
183-187	32.5	33.1	33.7	34.3	34.9	35.6	36.2	26.8	37.4
188-192	32.9	33.5	34.1	34.7	35.3	36.0	36.6	37.2	37.8
193-197	33.2	33.8	34.5	35.1	35.7	36.3	37.0	36.8	38.2
198-202	33.6	34.2	34.8	35.4	36.1	36.7	37.3	37.9	38.5
203-207	33.9	34.5	35.1	35.7	36.4	37.0	37.6	38.2	38.9

Source: Y's Way To Physical Fitness

PERCENT FAT ESTIMATE FOR WOMEN

Sum of Three Skinfolds

Triceps, Abdomen, Ilium

Sum of 3 Skinfolds	Age to Last Year								
	18 to 22	23 to 27	28 to 32	33 to 37	38 to 42	43 to 47	48 to 52	53 to 57	58 and older
8-12	8.8	9.0	9.2	9.4	9.5	9.7	9.9	10.1	10.3
13-17	10.8	10.9	11.1	11.3	11.5	11.7	11.8	12.0	12.2
18-22	12.6	12.8	13.0	13.2	13.4	13.5	13.7	13.9	14.1
23-27	14.5	14.6	14.8	15.0	15.2	15.4	15.6	15.7	15.9
28-32	16.2	16.4	16.6	16.8	17.0	17.1	17.3	17.5	17.7
33-37	17.9	18.1	18.3	18.5	18.7	18.9	19.0	19.2	19.4
38-42	19.6	19.8	20.0	20.2	20.3	20.5	20.7	20.9	21.1
43-47	21.2	21.4	21.6	21.8	21.9	22.1	22.3	22.5	22.7
48-52	22.8	22.9	23.1	23.3	23.5	23.7	23.8	24.0	24.2
53-57	24.2	24.4	24.6	24.8	25.0	25.2	25.3	25.5	25.7
									27.1
58-62	25.7	25.9	26.0	26.2	26.4	26.6	26.8	27.0	37.1
63-67	27.1	27.2	27.4	27.6	27.8	28.0	28.2	28.3	28.5
68-72	28.4	28.6	28.7	28.9	29.1	29.3	29.5	29.7	29.8
73-77	29.6	29.8	30.0	30.2	30.4	30.6	30.7	30.9	31.1
78-82	30.9	31.0	31.2	31.4	31.6	31.8	31.9	32.1	32.3
83-87	32.0	32.2	32.4	32.6	32.7	32.9	33.1	33.3	33.5
88-92	33.1	33.3	33.5	33.7	33.8	34.0	34.2	34.4	34.6
93-97	34.1	34.3	34.5	34.7	34.9	35.1	35.2	35.4	35.6
98-102	35.1	35.3	35.5	35.7	35.9	36.0	36.2	36.4	36.6
103-107	36.1	36.2	36.4	36.6	36.8	37.0	37.2	37.3	37.5
108-112	36.9	37.1	37.3	37.5	37.7	37.9	38.0	38.2	38.4
113-117	37.8	37.9	38.1	38.3	39.2	39.4	39.6	39.8	40.0
118-122	38.5	38.7	38.9	39.1	39.4	39.6	39.8	40.0	
123-127	39.2	39.4	39.6	39.8	40.0	40.1	40.3	40.5	40.7
128-132	39.9	40.1	40.2	40.4	40.6	40.8	41.0	41.2	41.3
133-137	40.5	40.7	40.8	41.0	41.2	41.4	41.6	41.7	41.9
138-142	41.0	41.2	41.4	41.6	41.7	41.9	42.1	42.3	42.5
143-147	41.5	41.7	41.9	42.0	42.2	42.4	42.6	42.8	43.0
148-152	41.9	42.1	42.3	42.8	42.6	42.8	43.0	43.2	43.4
153-157	42.3	42.5	42.6	52.8	43.0	43.2	43.4	43.6	43.7
158-162	42.6	42.8	42.0	43.1	43.3	43.5	43.7	43.9	44.1
163-167	42.9	43.0	43.2	43.4	43.6	43.8	44.0	44.1	44.3
168-172	43.1	43.2	43.4	43.6	43.8	44.0	44.2	44.3	44.5
173-177	43.2	43.4	43.6	43.8	43.9	44.1	44.3	44.5	44.7
178-182	43.3	43.5	43.7	43.8	44.0	44.2	44.4	44.6	44.8

APPENDIX B. CALORIC AND NUTRITIONAL VALUES OF FAST FOODS

	Wt (gm)	kcal	Pro* (gm)	Carb (gm)	Fat (gm)	Chol (mg)
BURGER CHEF						
Big Shef	186	542	23	35	34	—
Cheeseburger	104	304	14	24	17	—
Double Cheeseburger	145	434	24	24	26	—
French Fries	68	187	3	25	9	—
Hamburger, Regular	91	258	11	24	13	—
Mariner Platter	373	680	32	85	24	—
Rancher Platter	316	640	30	44	38	—
Shake	305	326	11	47	11	—
Skipper's Treat	179	604	21	47	37	—
Super Shef	252	600	29	39	37	—
BURGER KING						
Cheeseburger	—	305	17	29	13	—
Hamburger	—	252	14	29	9	—
Whopper	—	606	29	51	32	—
French Fries	—	214	3	28	10	—
Vanilla Shake	—	332	11	50	11	—
Whaler	—	486	18	64	46	—
Hot Dog	—	291	11	23	17	—
DAIRY QUEEN						
Big Brazier Deluxe	213	470	28	36	24	—
Big Brazier Regular	184	457	27	37	23	—
Big Brazier w/Cheese	213	553	32	38	30	—
Brazier w/Cheese	121	318	18	30	14	—
Brazier Cheese Dog	113	330	15	24	19	—
Brazier Chili Dog	128	330	13	25	20	—
Brazier Dog	99	273	11	23	15	—
Brazier French Fries, 2.5 oz	71	200	2	25	10	—
Brazier French Fries, 4.0 oz	113	320	3	40	16	—
Brazier Onion Rings	85	300	6	33	17	—
Brazier Regular	106	260	13	28	9	—
Fish Sandwich	170	400	20	41	17	—
Fish Sandwich w/Cheese	177	440	24	39	21	—
Super Brazier	298	783	53	35	48	—
Super Brazier Dog	182	518	20	41	30	—
Super Brazier Dog w/Cheese	203	593	26	43	36	—
Super Brazier Chili Dog	210	555	23	42	33	—
Banana Split	383	540	10	91	15	—
Buster Bar	149	390	10	37	22	—
DQ Chocolate Dipped Cone, sm	78	150	3	20	7	—
DQ Chocolate Dipped Cone, med	156	300	7	40	13	—
DQ Chocolate Dipped Cone, lg	234	450	10	58	20	—
DQ Chocolate Malt, sm	241	340	10	51	11	—
DQ Chocolate Malt, med	418	600	15	89	20	—
DQ Chocolate Malt, lg	588	840	22	125	28	—
DQ Chocolate Sundae, sm	106	170	4	30	4	—
DQ Chocolate Sundae, med	184	300	6	53	7	—
DQ Chocolate Sundae, lg	248	400	9	71	9	—
DQ Cone, sm	71	110	3	18	3	—
DQ Cone, med	142	230	6	35	7	—
DQ Cone, lg	213	340	10	52	10	—
Dairy Queen Parfait	284	460	10	81	11	—

CALORIC AND NUTRITIONAL VALUES OF FAST FOODS

	Wt (gm)	kcal	Pro* (gm)	Carb** (gm)	Fat (gm)	Chol† (mg)
Dilly Bar	85	240	4	22	15	—
DQ Float	397	330	6	59	8	—
DQ Freeze	397	520	11	89	13	—
DQ Sandwich	60	140	3	24	4	—
Fiesta Sundae	269	570	9	84	22	—
Hot Fudge Brownie Delight	266	570	11	83	22	—
Mr. Misty Float	404	440	6	85	8	—
Mr. Misty Freeze	411	500	10	87	12	—
KENTUCKY FRIED CHICKEN						
Individual Pieces						
(Original Recipe)						
Drumstick	54	136	14	2	8	73
Keel	96	283	25	6	13	90
Rib	82	241	19	8	15	97
Thigh	97	276	20	12	19	147
Wing	45	151	11	4	10	70
9 Pieces	652	1892	152	59	116	864
LONG JOHN SILVER'S						
Breaded Oysters, 6 pc	—	460	14	58	19	—
Breaded Clams, 5 oz	—	465	13	46	25	—
Chicken Planks, 4 pc	—	458	27	35	23	—
Cole Slaw, 4 oz	—	138	1	16	8	—
Corn on Cob, 1 pc	—	174	5	29	4	—
Fish w/Batter, 2 pc	—	318	19	19	19	—
Fish w/Batter, 3 pc	—	477	28	28	28	—
Fryes, 3 oz	—	275	4	32	15	—
Hush Puppies, 3 pc	—	153	1	20	7	—
Ocean Scallops, 6 pc	—	257	10	27	12	—
Peg Leg w/Batter, 5 pc	—	514	25	30	33	—
Shrimp w/Batter, 6 pc	—	269	9	31	13	—
Treasure Chest						
2 pc Fish, 2 Peg Legs	—	467	25	27	29	—
McDONALD'S						
Egg McMuffin	132	352	18	26	20	192
English Muffin, Buttered	62	186	6	28	6	12
Hot Cakes, w/Butter & Syrup	206	472	8	89	9	36
Sausage (Pork)	48	184	9	tr	17	43
Scrambled Eggs	77	162	12	2	12	301
Big Mac	187	541	26	39	31	75
Cheeseburger	114	306	16	31	13	41
Filet O Fish	131	402	15	34	23	43
French Fries	69	211	3	26	11	10
Hamburger	99	257	13	30	9	26
Quarter Pounder	164	418	26	33	21	69
Quarter Pounder w/Cheese	193	518	31	34	29	96
Apple Pie	91	300	2	31	19	14
Cherry Pie	92	298	2	33	18	14
McDonaldland Cookies	63	294	4	45	11	9
Chocolate Shake	289	364	11	60	9	29

CALORIC AND NUTRITIONAL VALUES OF FAST FOODS

	Wt (gm)	kcal	Pro* (gm)	Carb** (gm)	Fat (gm)	Chol† (mg)
Strawberry Shake	293	345	10	57	9	30
Vanilla Shake	289	323	10	52	8	29
PIZZA HUT						
Thin 'N Crispy						
Beef	—	490	29	51	19	—
Pork	—	520	27	51	23	—
Cheese	—	450	25	54	15	—
Pepperoni	—	430	23	45	17	—
Supreme	—	510	27	51	21	—
Thick 'N Chewy						
Beef	—	620	38	73	20	—
Pork	—	640	36	71	23	—
Cheese	—	560	34	71	14	—
Pepperoni	—	560	31	68	18	—
Supreme	—	640	36	74	22	—
TACO BELL						
Bean Burrito	166	343	11	48	12	—
Beef Burrito	184	466	30	37	21	—
Beefy Tostada	184	291	19	21	15	—
Bellbeefer	123	221	15	23	7	—
Bellbeefer w/Cheese	137	278	19	23	12	—
Burrito Supreme	225	457	21	43	22	—
Combination Burrito	175	404	21	43	16	—
Enchirito	207	454	25	42	21	—
Pintos 'N Cheese	158	168	11	21	5	—
Taco	83	186	15	14	8	—
Tostada	138	179	9	25	6	—
BEVERAGES						
Coffee, 6 oz	180	2	tr	tr	tr	—
Tea, 6 oz	180	2	tr	—	tr	—
Orange Juice, 6 oz	183	82	1	20	tr	—
Chocolate Milk, 8 oz	250	213	9	28	9	—
Skim Milk, 8 oz	245	88	9	13	tr	—
Whole Milk, 8 oz	244	159	9	12	9	27
Coca-Cola, 8 oz	246	96	0	24	0	—
Fanta Ginger Ale, 8 oz	244	84	0	21	0	—
Fanta Grape, 8 oz	247	114	0	29	0	—
Fanta Orange, 8 oz	248	117	0	30	0	—
Fanta Root Beer, 8 oz	246	103	0	27	0	—
Mr. Pibb, 8 oz	245	93	0	25	0	—
Mr. Pibb Without Sugar, 8 oz	237	1	0	tr	0	—
Sprite, 8 oz	245	95	0	24	0	—
Sprite Without Sugar, 8 oz	237	3	0	0	0	—
Tab, 8 oz	237	tr	0	tr	0	—
Fresca, 8 oz	237	2	0	0	0	—

*Protein.
**Carbohydrate.
†Cholesterol.

APPENDIX C. HIDDEN SUGAR (SUCROSE) IN FOODS

Approximate sugar content of popular foods in grams
(5 g = 1 tsp. = 20 calories)

Food		Serving	Sucrose (grams)
CANDY	Chocolate bar	1 average size	35
	Chocolate cream	1 average size	10
	Chocolate fudge	1½" sq. (15 to 1 lb.)	20
	Chocolate mints	1 medium (20 to 1 lb.)	15
	Marshmallow	1 average (60 to 1 lb.)	7
	Chewing gum	1 stick	3
CAKES AND COOKIES	Chocolate cake	1/12 cake (2 layer icing)	75
	Angel food cake	1/12 of large cake	30
	Sponge cake	1/10 of average cake	30
	Cream puff, iced	1 average custard filled	25
	Doughnut, plain	3" diameter	20
	Macaroons	1 large or 2 small	15
	Gingersnaps	1 medium	5
	Molasses cookies	3½" diameter	10
	Brownies	2" x 2" x ¾"	15
ICE CREAM	Ice cream	⅛ quart (½ cup)	30
	Sherbet	⅛ quart (½ cup)	40
PIE	Apple	1/6 med. pie	60
	Cherry	1/6 med. pie	70
	Raisin	1/6 med. pie	65
	Pumpkin	1/6 med. pie	50
SOFT DRINKS	Sweet carbonated beverage	1 bottle, 6 oz	22
	Ginger ale	6 oz. glass	18
MILK DRINKS	Chocolate	1 cup, 5 oz. milk	30
	Cocoa	1 cup, 5 oz. milk	20
	Eggnog	1 glass, 8 oz. milk	22

Food		Serving	Sucrose (grams)
SPREADS AND SAUCES	Jam	1 tbs. level	15
	Jelly	1 tbs. level	12
	Marmalade	1 tbs. level	15
	Syrup, maple	1 tbs. level	12
	Honey	1 tbs. level	15
	Chocolate sauce	1 tbs. thick	22
COOKED FRUITS	Peaches, canned in syrup	2 halves, 1 tbs. syrup	18
	Rhubarb, stewed, sweetened	½ cup	40
	Apple sauce, unsweetened	½ cup. scant	10
	Prunes, stewed, sweetened	4 to 5 med., 2 tbs. juice	40
DRIED FRUITS	Apricots, dried	4 to 6 halves	20
	Prunes, dried	3 to 4 medium	20
	Dates, dried	3 to 4 stoned	22
	Figs, dried	1½ to 2 small	20
	Raisins	¼ cup	20
FRUITS AND FRUIT JUICES	Fruit cocktail	½ cup. scant	25
	Orange juice	½ cup. scant	10
	Pineapple juice, unsweetened	½ cup. scant	13
	Grapefruit juice, unsweetened	½ cup. scant	11
	Grapefruit, commercial	½ cup. scant	18

SOURCE: Adapted from American Dental Association, *Diet and Dental Health.* 1967.

APPENDIX D. HIDDEN SALT IN FOODS

Sodium in Processed Foods

Product	Amount	Sodium (mg)
Pepperidge Farm White Bread	2 slices	234
Wonder Enriched Bread	2 slices	355
Pepperidge Farm Whole Wheat Bread	2 slices	214
Kellogg's Corn Flakes	1 ounce	320
Kellogg's Sugar Frosted Flakes	1 ounce	186
Campbell's Tomato Soup	10-ounce serving	1050
Campbell's Tomato Juice	8 ounces	744
Lipton Vegetable Cup-a-Soup	8 ounces	1058
Breakstone's Lowfat Cottage Cheese	½ cup	435
Kraft Processed American Cheese	1 ounce	238
Kraft Cheddar Cheese	1 ounce	190
Morton King Size Turkey Dinner	1 dinner	2567
Swanson Fried Chicken Dinner	1 dinner	1152
Swanson Turkey Dinner	1 dinner	1735
Campbell's Beans & Franks	8 ounces	958
Oscar Mayer Beef Franks	1 frank	425
Chef Boyardee Beefaroni	7.5 ounces	1186
B&M Brick Oven Baked Beans	1 cup	810
Del Monte Whole Green Beans	1 cup	925
McDonald's Big Mac	1	1510
Burger King Whopper	1	909
Arthur Treacher's Fish Sandwich	1	836
Kentucky Fried Chicken Dinner original recipe (3 pieces chicken)	1	2285
Nabisco Premium Saltines	10 (1 ounce)	430
Mister Salty Very Thin Pretzel Sticks	1 ounce	735
Heinz Kosher Dill Pickles	1 large	1137
Heinz Mustard	1 tablespoon	212
Heinz Tomato Ketchup	1 tablespoon	154
Jell-O Chocolate Flavor Instant Pudding & Pie Filling	½ cup	480
Hostess Twinkies	1	190
Pillsbury Chocolate Chip Cookies	3	140
Nabisco Oreo Sandwich Cookies	3	240

Note: Based on analyses by Consumers Union, the Center for Science in the Public Interests, and manufacturers.

Salt in Natural Foods and in Processed Foods

Food	Portion	Sodium content
Salmon, fresh	3 oz.	99 milligrams
Salmon, canned without salt added	3 oz.	41 milligrams
Salmon canned, salt added	3 oz.	443 milligrams
Tuna, canned, low sodium	3 oz.	34 milligrams
Tuna, canned	3 oz.	303 milligrams
Shrimp, fresh	3 oz.	137 milligrams
Shrimp, canned	3 oz.	1,955 milligrams
Swiss cheese	1 oz.	74 milligrams
Swiss cheese style "food"	1 oz.	440 milligrams
Cottage cheese, unsalted	1 oz.	14 milligrams
Cottage cheese, salted	1 oz.	457 milligrams
Beef, lean	3 oz.	55 milligrams
Dried beef, chipped	3 oz.	1,219 milligrams
Frankfurter	1 frank	639 milligrams
Liver	3 oz.	33 milligrams
Braunschweiger	1 slice	324 milligrams
Oatmeal	3/4 cup	1 milligram
Oatmeal, instant, salt added	3/4 cup	283 milligrams
Rice Crispies	1 cup	340 milligrams
Macaroni	1 cup	2 milligrams
Macaroni and beef, canned	1 cup	1,185 milligrams
Beans, lima	1 cup	3 milligrams
Beans, lima, canned	1 cup	465 milligrams
Soy sauce	1 tbsp	1,029 milligrams

APPENDIX E. CALORIES FROM CONDIMENTS

Condiments can fool you — some have as many or more calories than the foods we put them on. Many also are high in fat and therefore should be avoided as much as possible.

Check the list below and see if the calories you are getting are worth it.

Condiment	Calories Per Tbsp.	Condiment	Calories Per Tbsp.
Vegetable Oil	120	Sugar	46
Butter	102	Cream (light)	32
Margarine	102	Barbecue Sauce	23
Mayonnaise	101	Pickle Relish (sweet)	21
Tartar sauce	74	Steak sauce	21
Honey	64	Catsup	16
Maple Syrup	60	Mustard	15
Jams and Preserves	54	Worchestershire sauce	12
Cream Cheese	52		

APPENDIX F. NUTRITIVE VALUES OF FOODS

The following charts are from the publication *Nutritive Value of Foods* published by the United States Department of Agriculture.

Key to Abbreviations

A Item Number (for reference)

B Food, approximate measures, units, and weight
(edible part unless indicated otherwise in footnotes)

C Water (percent)

D Food energy (calories)

E Protein (grams)

F Fat (grams)

G Fatty Acids: Saturated (total in grams)

H Fatt Acids: Unsaturated — Oleic (grams)

I Fatty Acids: Unsaturated — Linoleic (grams)

J Carbohydrates (grams)

K Calcium (milligrams)

L Phosphorus (milligrams)

M Iron (milligrams)

N Potassium (milligrams)

O Vitamin A value (international units)

P Thiamine (milligrams)

Q Riboflavin (milligrams)

R Niacin (milligrams)

S Ascorbic acid (milligrams)

DAIRY PRODUCTS (CHEESE, CREAM, IMITATION CREAM, MILK, RELATED PRODUCTS)

Butter. See Fats, oils; related products, items 103-108.

(A)	(B)	(C) Grams	(C) per cent	(D) Cal-ories	(E) Grams	(F) Grams	(G) Grams	(H) Grams	(I) Grams	(J) Grams	(K) Milli-grams	(L) Milli-grams	(M) Milli-grams	(N) Milli-grams	(O) Inter-national units	(P) Milli-grams	(Q) Milli-grams	(R) Milli-grams	(S) Milli-grams
	Cheese:																		
	Natural:																		
1	Blue — 1 oz	28	42	100	6	8	5.3	1.9	0.2	1	150	110	0.1	73	200	0.01	0.11	0.3	0
2	Camembert (3 wedges per 4-oz container) — 1 wedge	38	52	115	8	9	5.8	2.2	.2	Trace	147	132	.1	71	350	.01	.19	.2	0
	Cheddar:																		
3	Cut pieces — 1 oz	28	37	115	7	9	6.1	2.1	.2	Trace	204	145	.2	28	300	.01	.11	Trace	0
4	1 cu in	17.2	37	70	4	6	3.7	1.3	.1	Trace	124	88	.1	17	180	Trace	.06	Trace	0
5	Shredded — 1 cup	113	37	455	28	37	24.2	8.5	.7	1	815	579	.8	111	1,200	.03	.42	.1	0
	Cottage (curd not pressed down):																		
	Creamed (cottage cheese, 4% fat):																		
6	Large curd — 1 cup	225	79	235	28	10	6.4	2.4	.2	6	135	297	.3	190	370	.05	.37	.3	Trace
7	Small curd — 1 cup	210	79	220	26	9	6.0	2.2	.2	6	126	277	.3	177	340	.04	.34	.3	Trace
8	Low fat (2%) — 1 cup	226	79	205	31	4	2.8	1.0	.1	8	155	340	.4	217	160	.05	.42	.3	Trace
9	Low fat (1%) — 1 cup	226	82	165	28	2	1.5	.5	.1	6	138	302	.3	193	80	.05	.37	.3	Trace
10	Uncreamed (cottage cheese dry curd, less than 1/2% fat) — 1 cup	145	80	125	25	1	.4	.1	Trace	3	46	151	.3	47	40	.04	.21	.2	0
11	Cream — 1 oz	28	54	100	2	10	6.2	2.4	.2	1	23	30	.3	34	400	Trace	.06	Trace	0
	Mozzarella, made with—																		
12	Whole milk — 1 oz	28	48	90	6	7	4.4	1.7	.2	1	163	117	.1	21	260	Trace	.08	Trace	0
13	Part skim milk — 1 oz	28	49	80	8	5	3.1	1.2	.1	1	207	149	.1	27	180	.01	.10	Trace	0
	Parmesan, grated:																		
14	Cup, not pressed down — 1 cup	100	18	455	42	30	19.1	7.7	.3	4	1,376	807	1.0	107	700	.05	.39	.3	0
15	Tablespoon — 1 tbsp	5	18	25	2	2	1.0	.4	Trace	Trace	69	40	Trace	5	40	Trace	.02	Trace	0
16	Ounce — 1 oz	28	18	130	12	9	5.4	2.2	.1	1	390	229	.3	30	200	.01	.11	Trace	0
17	Provolone — 1 oz	28	41	100	7	8	4.8	1.7	.1	1	214	141	.1	39	230	.01	.09	Trace	0
	Ricotta, made with—																		
18	Whole milk — 1 cup	246	72	428	28	32	20.4	7.1	.7	7	509	389	.9	257	1,210	.03	.48	.3	0
19	Part skim milk — 1 cup	246	74	340	28	19	12.1	4.7	.5	13	669	449	1.1	308	1,060	.05	.46	.2	0
20	Romano — 1 oz	28	31	110	9	8					302	215			160				0
21	Swiss — 1 oz	28	37	105	8	8	5.0	1.7	.2	1	272	171	Trace	31	240	.01	.10	Trace	0
	Pasteurized process cheese:																		
22	American — 1 oz	28	39	105	6	9	5.6	2.1	.2	Trace	174	211	.1	46	340	.01	.10	Trace	0
23	Swiss — 1 oz	28	42	95	7	7	4.5	1.7	.1	1	219	216	.2	61	230	Trace	.08	Trace	0
24	Pasteurized process cheese food, American — 1 oz	28	43	95	6	7	4.4	1.7	.2	2	163	130	.2	79	260	.01	.13	Trace	0
25	Pasteurized process cheese spread, American — 1 oz	28	48	82	5	6	3.8	1.5	.1	2	159	202	.1	69	220	.01	.12	Trace	0
	Cream, sweet:																		
26	Half-and-half (cream and milk) — 1 cup	242	81	315	7	28	17.3	7.0	.6	10	254	230	.2	314	260	.08	.36	.2	2
27	1 tbsp	15	81	20	Trace	2	1.1	.4	Trace	1	16	14	Trace	19	20	.01	.02	Trace	Trace
28	Light, coffee, or table — 1 cup	240	74	470	6	46	28.8	11.7	1.0	9	231	192	.1	292	1,730	.08	.36	.1	2
29	1 tbsp	15	74	30	Trace	3	1.8	.7	.1	1	14	12	Trace	18	110	Trace	.02	Trace	Trace

(A)	(B) Foods, approximate measures, units, and weight	(C) grams	(D) Water %	(E) Food energy (Cal)	(F) Protein (g)	(G) Fat (g)	(H) Sat. (g)	(I) Oleic (g)	(J) Linoleic (g)	(K) Carbohydrate (g)	(L) Calcium (mg)	(M) Phosphorus (mg)	(N) Iron (mg)	(O) Potassium (mg)	(P) Vit. A (I.U.)	(Q) Thiamin (mg)	(R) Riboflavin (mg)	(S) Niacin (mg)	(T) Ascorbic acid (mg)
	Whipping, unwhipped (volume about double when whipped):																		
30	Light — 1 cup	239	64	700	5	74	46.2	18.3	1.5	7	166	146	0.1	231	2,690	0.06	0.30	0.1	1
31	— 1 tbsp	15	64	45	Trace	5	2.9	1.1	.1	Trace	10	9	Trace	15	170	Trace	.02	Trace	Trace
32	Heavy — 1 cup	238	58	820	5	88	54.8	22.2	2.0	7	154	149	.1	179	3,500	.05	.26	.1	1
33	— 1 tbsp	15	58	80	Trace	6	3.5	1.4	.1	Trace	10	9	Trace	11	220	Trace	.02	Trace	Trace
34	Whipped topping, (pressurized) — 1 cup	60	61	155	2	13	8.3	3.4	.3	7	61	54	Trace	88	550	.02	.04	Trace	0
35	— 1 tbsp	3	61	10	Trace	1	.4	.2	Trace	Trace	3	3	Trace	4	30	Trace	Trace	Trace	0
36	Cream, sour — 1 cup	230	71	495	7	48	30.0	12.1	1.1	10	268	195	.1	331	1,820	.08	.34	.2	2
37	— 1 tbsp	12	71	25	Trace	3	1.6	.6	.1	1	14	10	Trace	17	90	Trace	.02	Trace	Trace
	Cream products, imitation (made with vegetable fat):																		
	Sweet:																		
	Creamers:																		
38	Liquid (frozen) — 1 cup	245	77	335	2	24	22.8	.3	Trace	28	23	157	.1	467	220[40]	0	0	0	0
39	— 1 tbsp	15	77	20	Trace	1	1.4	Trace	0	2	1	10	Trace	29	10[40]	0	0	0	0
40	Powdered — 1 cup	94	2	515	5	33	30.6	.9	Trace	52	21	397	.1	763	190[40]	0	.16[40]	0	0
41	— 1 tsp	2	2	10	Trace	1	.7	Trace	0	1	Trace	8	Trace	16	Trace[40]	0	Trace[40]	0	0
	Whipped topping:																		
42	Frozen — 1 cup	75	50	240	1	19	16.3	1.0	.2	17	5	6	.1	14	650[40]	0	0	0	0
43	— 1 tbsp	4	50	15	Trace	1	.9	.1	Trace	1	Trace	Trace	Trace	1	30[40]	0	0	0	0
44	Powdered, made with whole milk — 1 cup	80	67	150	3	10	8.5	.7	.2	13	72	69	Trace	121	290[40]	.02	.09	Trace	1
45	— 1 tbsp	4	67	10	Trace	Trace	.4	Trace	Trace	1	4	3	Trace	6	10[40]	Trace	Trace	Trace	Trace
46	Pressurized — 1 cup	70	60	185	1	16	13.2	1.4	.2	11	4	13	Trace	13	330[40]	0	0	0	0
47	— 1 tbsp	4	60	10	Trace	1	.8	.1	Trace	1	Trace	1	Trace	1	20[40]	0	0	0	0
48	Sour dressing (imitation sour cream) made with nonfat dry milk — 1 cup	235	75	415	8	39	31.2	4.4	1.1	11	266	205	.1	380	20[40]	.09	.38	.2	2
49	— 1 tbsp	12	75	20	Trace	2	1.6	.2	.1	1	14	10	Trace	19	Trace[40]	.01	.02	Trace	Trace
	Ice cream. See Milk desserts, frozen (items 75–80).																		
	Ice milk. See Milk desserts, frozen (items 81–83).																		
	Milk:																		
	Fluid:																		
50	Whole (3.3% fat) — 1 cup	244	88	150	8	8	5.1	2.1	.2	11	291	228	.1	370	310	.09	.40	.2	2
	Lowfat (2%):																		
51	No milk solids added — 1 cup	244	89	120	8	5	2.9	1.2	.1	12	297	232	.1	377	500[41]	.10	.40	.2	2
	Milk solids added:																		
52	Label claim less than 10 g of protein per cup — 1 cup	245	89	125	9	5	2.9	1.2	.1	12	313	245	.1	397	500[41]	.10	.42	.2	2
53	Label claim 10 or more grams of protein per cup (protein fortified) — 1 cup	246	88	135	10	5	3.0	1.2	.1	14	352	276	.1	447	500[41]	.11	.48	.2	3
	Lowfat (1%):																		
54	No milk solids added — 1 cup	244	90	100	8	3	1.6	.7	.1	12	300	235	.1	381	500[41]	.10	.41	.2	2
	Milk solids added:																		
55	Label claim less than 10 g of protein per cup — 1 cup	245	90	105	9	2	1.5	.6	.1	12	313	245	.1	397	500[41]	.10	.42	.2	2
56	Label claim 10 or more grams of protein per cup (protein fortified) — 1 cup	246	89	120	10	3	1.8	.7	.1	14	349	273	.1	444	500[41]	.11	.47	.2	3
	Nonfat (skim):																		
57	No milk solids added — 1 cup	245	91	85	8	Trace	.3	.1	Trace	12	302	247	.1	406	500[41]	.09	.37	.2	2

[40] Vitamin A value is largely from beta-carotene used for coloring. Riboflavin value for items 40–41 apply to products with added riboflavin.

[41] Applies to product without added vitamin A. With added vitamin A, value is 500 International Units (I.U.).

DAIRY PRODUCTS (CHEESE, CREAM, IMITATION CREAM, MILK, RELATED PRODUCTS)—Con.

(A)	(B)	(C) Grams	(C) Per-cent	(D) Cal-ories	(E) Grams	(F) Grams	(G) Grams	(H) Grams	(I) Grams	(J) Grams	(K) Milli-grams	(L) Milli-grams	(M) Milli-grams	(N) Milli-grams	(O) Inter-national units	(P) Milli-grams	(Q) Milli-grams	(R) Milli-grams	(S) Milli-grams
	Milk—Continued																		
	Fluid—Continued																		
	Nonfat (skim)—Continued																		
	Milk solids added:																		
58	Label claim less than 10 g of protein per cup. 1 cup	245	90	90	9	1	0.4	0.1	Trace	12	316	255	0.1	418	500	0.10	0.43	0.2	2
59	Label claim 10 or more grams of protein per cup (protein fortified). 1 cup	246	89	100	10	1	.4	.1	Trace	14	352	275	.1	446	500	.11	.48	.2	3
60	Buttermilk 1 cup	245	90	100	8	2	1.3	.5	Trace	12	285	219	.1	371	980	.08	.38	.1	2
	Canned:																		
	Evaporated, unsweetened:																		
61	Whole milk 1 cup	252	74	340	17	19	11.6	5.3	0.4	25	657	510	.5	764	[5]610	.12	.80	.5	5
62	Skim milk 1 cup	255	79	200	19	1	.3	.1	Trace	29	738	497	.7	845	[5]1,000	.11	.79	.4	3
63	Sweetened, condensed 1 cup	306	27	980	24	27	16.8	6.7	.7	166	868	775	.6	1,136	[5]1,000	.28	1.27	.6	8
	Dried:																		
64	Buttermilk 1 cup	120	3	465	41	7	4.3	1.7	.2	59	1,421	1,119	.4	1,910	[5]260	.47	1.90	1.1	7
	Nonfat instant:																		
65	Envelope, net wt., 3.2 oz. 1 envelope	91	4	325	32	1	.4	.1	Trace	47	1,120	896	.3	1,552	[6]2,160	.38	1.59	.8	5
66	1 cup	68	4	245	24	Trace	.3	.1	Trace	35	837	670	.2	1,160	[6]1,610	.28	1.19	.6	4
	Milk beverages:																		
	Chocolate milk (commercial):																		
67	Regular 1 cup	250	82	210	8	8	5.3	2.2	.2	26	280	251	.6	417	300	.09	.41	.3	2
68	Lowfat (2%) 1 cup	250	84	180	8	5	3.1	1.3	.1	26	284	254	.6	422	500	.10	.42	.3	2
69	Lowfat (1%) 1 cup	250	85	160	8	3	1.5	.7	.1	26	287	257	.6	426	500	.10	.40	.2	2
70	Eggnog (commercial) 1 cup	254	74	340	10	19	11.3	5.0	.6	34	330	278	.5	420	890	.09	.48	.3	4
	Malted milk, home-prepared with 1 cup of whole milk and 2 to 3 heaping tsp of malted milk powder (about 3/4 oz):																		
71	Chocolate 1 cup of milk plus 3/4 oz of powder.	265	81	235	9	9	5.5	—	—	29	304	265	.5	500	330	.14	.43	.7	2
72	Natural 1 cup of milk plus 3/4 oz of powder.	265	81	235	11	10	6.0	—	—	27	347	307	.3	529	380	.20	.54	1.3	2
	Shakes, thick:[8]																		
73	Chocolate, container, net wt., 10.6 oz. 1 container	300	72	355	9	8	5.0	2.0	.2	63	396	378	.9	672	260	.14	.67	.4	0
74	Vanilla, container, net wt. 11 oz. 1 container	313	74	350	12	9	5.9	2.4	.2	56	457	361	.3	572	360	.09	.61	.5	0
	Milk desserts, frozen:																		
	Ice cream:																		
	Regular (about 11% fat):																		
75	Hardened 1/2 gal	1,064	61	2,155	38	115	71.3	28.8	2.6	254	1,406	1,075	1.0	2,052	4,340	.42	2.63	1.1	6
76	1 cup	133	61	270	5	14	8.9	3.6	.3	32	176	134	.1	257	540	.05	.33	.1	1
77	3-fl oz container	50	61	100	2	5	3.4	1.4	.1	12	66	51	Trace	96	200	.02	.12	.1	Trace
78	Soft serve (frozen custard) 1 cup	173	60	375	7	23	13.5	5.9	.6	38	236	199	.4	338	790	.08	.45	.2	1
79	Rich (about 16% fat), hardened. 1/2 gal	1,188	59	2,805	33	190	118.3	47.8	4.3	256	1,213	927	.8	1,771	7,200	.36	2.27	.9	5
80	1 cup	148	59	350	4	24	14.7	6.0	.5	32	151	115	.1	221	900	.04	.28	.1	1
	Ice milk:																		
	Hardened (about 4.3% fat)																		
81	1/2 gal	1,048	69	1,470	41	45	28.1	11.3	1.0	232	1,409	1,035	1.5	2,117	1,710	.61	2.78	.9	6
82	1 cup	131	69	185	5	6	3.5	1.4	.1	29	176	129	.1	265	210	.08	.35	.1	1

(A)	(B)	(C)	(D)	(E)	(F)	(G)	(H)	(I)	(J)	(K)	(L)	(M)	(N)	(O)	(P)	(Q)	(R)	(S)
83	Soft serve (about 2.6% fat)------- 1 cup — 175	70	225	8	5	2.9	1.2	0.1	38	274	202	0.3	412	180	0.12	0.54	0.2	1
84	Sherbet (about 2% fat): ----------- 1/2 gal — 1,542	66	2,160	17	31	19.0	7.7	.7	469	827	594	2.5	1,585	1,480	.26	.71	.1	31
85	------- 1 cup — 193	66	270	2	4	2.4	1.0	.1	59	103	74	.3	198	190	.03	.09	.1	4
86	Custard, baked------- 1 cup — 265	77	305	14	15	6.8	5.4	.7	29	297	310	1.1	387	930	.11	.50	.3	1
	Puddings:																	
	From home recipe:																	
	Starch base:																		
87	Chocolate------- 1 cup — 260	66	385	8	12	7.6	3.3	.3	67	250	255	1.3	445	390	.05	.36	.3	1
88	Vanilla (blancmange)------- 1 cup — 255	76	285	9	10	6.2	2.5	.2	41	298	232	Trace	352	410	.08	.41	.3	2
89	Tapioca cream------- 1 cup — 165	72	220	8	8	4.1	2.5	.5	28	173	180	.7	223	480	.07	.30	.2	2
	From mix (chocolate) and milk:																	
90	Regular (cooked)------- 1 cup — 260	70	320	9	8	4.3	2.6	.2	59	265	247	.8	354	340	.05	.39	.3	2
91	Instant------- 1 cup — 260	69	325	8	7	3.6	2.2	.3	63	374	237	1.3	335	340	.08	.39	.3	2
	Yogurt:																		
	With added milk solids:																		
	Made with lowfat milk:																		
92	Fruit-flavored------- 1 container, net wt., 8 oz — 227	75	230	10	3	1.8	.6	.1	42	343	269	.2	439	[10]120	.08	.40	.2	1
93	Plain------- 1 container, net wt., 8 oz — 227	85	145	12	4	2.3	.8	.1	16	415	326	.2	531	[10]150	.10	.49	.3	2
94	Made with nonfat milk------- 1 container, net wt., 8 oz — 227	85	125	13	Trace	.3	.1	Trace	17	452	355	.2	579	[10]120	.11	.53	.3	2
	Without added milk solids:																		
95	Made with whole milk------- 1 container, net wt., 8 oz — 227	88	140	8	7	4.8	1.7	.1	11	274	215	.1	351	280	.07	.32	.2	1
	EGGS																		
	Eggs, large (24 oz per dozen):																		
	Raw:																		
96	Whole, without shell------- 1 egg — 50	75	85	6	6	1.7	2.0	.6	1	28	90	1.0	65	260	.04	.15	Trace	0
97	White------- 1 white — 33	88	15	3	Trace	0	0	0	Trace	4	4	Trace	45	0	Trace	.09	Trace	0
98	Yolk------- 1 yolk — 17	49	65	3	6	1.7	2.1	.6	Trace	26	86	.9	15	310	.04	.07	Trace	0
	Cooked:																		
99	Fried in butter------- 1 egg — 46	72	85	5	6	2.4	2.2	.6	1	26	80	.9	58	290	.03	.13	Trace	0
100	Hard-cooked, shell removed------- 1 egg — 50	75	80	6	6	1.7	2.0	.6	1	28	90	1.0	65	260	.04	.14	Trace	0
101	Poached------- 1 egg — 50	74	80	6	5	1.7	2.0	.6	1	28	90	1.0	65	260	.04	.13	Trace	0
102	Scrambled (milk added) in butter. Also omelet------- 1 egg — 64	76	95	6	7	2.8	2.3	.6	1	47	97	.9	85	310	.04	.16	Trace	0
	FATS, OILS; RELATED PRODUCTS																		
	Butter:																		
	Regular (1 brick or 4 sticks per lb):																		
103	Stick (1/2 cup)------- 1 stick — 113	16	815	1	92	57.3	23.1	2.1	Trace	27	26	.2	29	[11]3,470	.01	.04	Trace	0
104	Tablespoon (about 1/8 stick)------- 1 tbsp — 14	16	100	Trace	12	7.2	2.9	.3	Trace	3	3	Trace	4	[11]430	Trace	Trace	Trace	0
105	Pat (1 in square, 1/3 in high; 90 per lb)------- 1 pat — 5	16	35	Trace	4	2.5	1.0	.1	Trace	1	1	Trace	1	[11]150	Trace	Trace	Trace	0
	Whipped (6 sticks or two 8-oz containers per lb):																		
106	Stick (1/2 cup)------- 1 stick — 76	16	540	1	61	38.2	15.4	1.4	Trace	18	17	.1	20	[12]2,310	Trace	.03	Trace	0
107	Tablespoon (about 1/8 stick)------- 1 tbsp — 9	16	65	Trace	8	4.7	1.9	.2	Trace	2	2	Trace	2	[11]290	Trace	Trace	Trace	0
108	Pat (1 1/4 in square, 1/3 in high; 120 per lb)------- 1 pat — 4	16	25	Trace	3	1.9	.8	.1	Trace	1	1	Trace	1	[11]120	0	Trace	Trace	0

[3] Applies to product without vitamin A added.
[4] Applies to product with added vitamin A. Without added vitamin A, value is 20 International Units (I.U.).
[5] Yields 1 qt of fluid milk when reconstituted according to package directions.
[6] Applies to product with added vitamin A.
[7] Weight applies to product with label claim of 1 1/3 cups equal 3.2 oz.
[8] Applies to products made from thick shake mixes and that do not contain added ice cream. Products made from milk shake mixes are higher in fat and usually contain added ice cream.
[9] Content of fat, vitamin A, and carbohydrate varies. Consult the label when precise values are needed for special diets.
[10] Applies to product made with milk containing no added vitamin A.
[11] Based on year-round average.

FATS, OILS; RELATED PRODUCTS—Con.

(A)	(B)		(C)	(D)	(E)	(F)	(G)	(H)	(I)	(J)	(K)	(L)	(M)	(N)	(O)	(P)	(Q)	(R)	(S)
		Grams	Per cent	Calories	Grams	Grams	Grams	Grams	Grams	Grams	Milligrams	Milligrams	Milligrams	Milligrams	International units	Milligrams	Milligrams	Milligrams	Milligrams
109	Fats, cooking (vegetable shortenings). — 1 cup	200	0	1,770	0	200	48.8	88.2	48.4	0	0	0	0	0	—	0	0	0	0
110	— 1 tbsp	13	0	110	0	13	3.2	5.7	3.1	0	0	0	0	0	—	0	0	0	0
111	Lard — 1 cup	205	0	1,850	0	205	81.0	83.8	20.5	0	0	0	0	0	0	0	0	0	0
112	— 1 tbsp	13	0	115	0	13	5.1	5.3	1.3	0	0	0	0	0	0	0	0	0	0
	Margarine: Regular (1 brick or 4 sticks per lb):																		
113	Stick (1/2 cup) — 1 stick	113	16	815	1	92	16.7	42.9	24.9	Trace	27	26	.2	29	[12]3,750	.01	.04	Trace	0
114	Tablespoon (about 1/8 stick) — 1 tbsp	14	16	100	Trace	12	2.1	5.3	3.1	Trace	3	3	Trace	4	[12]470	Trace	Trace	Trace	0
115	Pat (1 in square, 1/3 in high; 90 per lb) — 1 pat	5	16	35	Trace	4	.7	1.9	1.1	Trace	1	1	Trace	1	[12]170	Trace	Trace	Trace	0
116	Soft, two 8-oz containers per lb. — 1 container	227	16	1,635	1	184	32.5	71.5	65.4	Trace	53	52	.4	59	[12]7,500	.01	.08	.1	0
117	— 1 tbsp	14	16	100	Trace	12	2.0	4.5	4.1	Trace	3	3	Trace	4	[12]470	Trace	Trace	Trace	0
	Whipped (6 sticks per lb):																		
118	Stick (1/2 cup) — 1 stick	76	16	545	Trace	61	11.2	28.7	16.7	Trace	18	17	.1	20	[12]2,500	Trace	.03	Trace	0
119	Tablespoon (about 1/8 stick) — 1 tbsp	9	16	70	Trace	8	1.4	3.6	2.1	Trace	2	2	Trace	2	[12]310	Trace	Trace	Trace	0
	Oils, salad or cooking:																		
120	Corn — 1 cup	218	0	1,925	0	218	27.7	53.6	125.1	0	0	0	0	0	—	0	0	0	0
121	— 1 tbsp	14	0	120	0	14	1.7	3.3	7.8	0	0	0	0	0	—	0	0	0	0
122	Olive — 1 cup	216	0	1,910	0	216	30.7	154.4	17.1	0	0	0	0	0	—	0	0	0	0
123	— 1 tbsp	14	0	120	0	14	1.9	9.7	1.1	0	0	0	0	0	—	0	0	0	0
124	Peanut — 1 cup	216	0	1,910	0	216	37.4	98.5	67.0	0	0	0	0	0	—	0	0	0	0
125	— 1 tbsp	14	0	120	0	14	2.3	6.2	4.2	0	0	0	0	0	—	0	0	0	0
126	Safflower — 1 cup	218	0	1,925	0	218	20.5	25.9	159.8	0	0	0	0	0	—	0	0	0	0
127	— 1 tbsp	14	0	120	0	14	1.3	1.6	10.0	0	0	0	0	0	—	0	0	0	0
128	Soybean oil, hydrogenated (partially hardened) — 1 cup	218	0	1,925	0	218	31.8	93.1	75.6	0	0	0	0	0	—	0	0	0	0
129	— 1 tbsp	14	0	120	0	14	2.0	5.8	4.7	0	0	0	0	0	—	0	0	0	0
130	Soybean-cottonseed oil blend, hydrogenated. — 1 cup	218	0	1,925	0	218	38.2	63.0	99.6	0	0	0	0	0	—	0	0	0	0
131	— 1 tbsp	14	0	120	0	14	2.4	3.9	6.2	0	0	0	0	0	—	0	0	0	0
	Salad dressings: Commercial: Blue cheese:																		
132	Regular — 1 tbsp	15	32	75	1	8	1.6	1.7	3.8	1	12	11	Trace	6	30	Trace	.02	Trace	Trace
133	Low calorie (5 Cal per tsp) — 1 tbsp	16	84	10	1	1	.5	.3	Trace	1	10	8	Trace	5	30	Trace	.01	Trace	Trace
	French:																		
134	Regular — 1 tbsp	16	39	65	Trace	6	1.1	1.3	3.2	3	2	2	.1	13	—	—	—	—	—
135	Low calorie (5 Cal per tsp) — 1 tbsp	16	77	15	Trace	Trace	.1	.1	.4	2	2	2	.1	13	—	—	—	—	—
	Italian:																		
136	Regular — 1 tbsp	15	28	85	Trace	9	1.6	1.9	4.7	1	2	1	Trace	2	Trace	Trace	Trace	Trace	—
137	Low calorie (2 Cal per tsp) — 1 tbsp	15	90	10	Trace	Trace	.1	.1	.1	Trace	2	1	Trace	2	Trace	Trace	Trace	Trace	—
138	Mayonnaise — 1 tbsp	14	15	100	Trace	11	2.0	2.4	5.6	Trace	3	4	.1	5	40	Trace	.01	Trace	—
	Mayonnaise type:																		
139	Regular — 1 tbsp	15	41	65	Trace	6	1.1	1.4	3.2	2	2	4	Trace	1	30	Trace	Trace	Trace	—
140	Low calorie (8 Cal per tsp) — 1 tbsp	16	81	20	Trace	2	.4	.4	1.0	2	3	4	Trace	1	40	Trace	Trace	Trace	—
141	Tartar sauce, regular — 1 tbsp	14	34	75	Trace	8	1.5	1.8	4.1	1	3	4	.1	11	30	Trace	Trace	Trace	Trace
	Thousand Island:																		
142	Regular — 1 tbsp	16	32	80	Trace	8	1.4	1.7	4.0	2	2	3	.1	18	50	Trace	Trace	Trace	Trace
143	Low calorie (10 Cal per tsp) — 1 tbsp	15	68	25	Trace	2	.4	.4	1.0	2	2	3	.1	17	50	Trace	Trace	Trace	Trace
144	From home recipe: Cooked type — 1 tbsp	16	68	25	1	2	.5	.6	.3	2	14	15	.1	19	80	.01	.03	Trace	Trace

FISH, SHELLFISH, MEAT, POULTRY; RELATED PRODUCTS

(A)	(B)	(C)	(D)	(E)	(F)	(G)	(H)	(I)	(J)	(K)	(L)	(M)	(N)	(O)	(P)	(Q)	(R)	(S)
	Fish and shellfish:																	
145	Bluefish, baked with butter or margarine — 3 oz	85	135	22	4	—	—	—	0	25	244	0.6	—	40	0.09	0.08	1.6	—
	Clams:																	
146	Raw, meat only — 3 oz	85	65	11	1	—	Trace	—	2	59	138	5.2	154	90	0.08	0.15	1.1	8
147	Canned, solids and liquid — 3 oz	85	45	7	1	0.2	Trace	—	2	47	116	3.5	119	—	0.01	0.09	0.9	—
148	Crabmeat (white or king), canned, not pressed down — 1 cup	135	135	24	3	0.6	0.4	0.1	1	61	246	1.1	149	—	0.11	0.11	2.6	—
149	Fish sticks, breaded, cooked, frozen (stick, 4 by 1 by 1/2 in) — 1 fish stick or 1 oz	28	50	5	3	—	—	—	2	3	47	0.1	—	0	0.01	0.02	0.5	—
150	Haddock, breaded, fried[15] — 3 oz	85	140	17	5	1.4	2.2	1.2	5	34	210	1.0	296	—	0.03	0.06	2.7	2
151	Ocean perch, breaded, fried[15] — 1 fillet	85	195	16	11	2.7	4.4	2.3	6	28	192	1.1	242	—	0.10	0.10	1.6	—
152	Oysters, raw, meat only (13-19 medium Selects) — 1 cup	240	160	20	4	1.3	0.2	0.1	8	226	343	13.2	290	740	0.34	0.43	6.0	—
153	Salmon, pink, canned, solids and liquid — 3 oz	85	120	17	5	0.9	0.8	0.1	0	[16]167	243	0.7	307	60	0.03	0.16	6.8	—
154	Sardines, Atlantic, canned in oil, drained solids — 3 oz	85	175	20	9	3.0	2.5	0.5	0	372	424	2.5	502	190	0.02	0.17	4.6	—
155	Scallops, frozen, breaded, fried, reheated — 6 scallops	90	175	16	8	—	—	—	9	—	—	—	—	—	—	—	—	—
156	Shad, baked with butter or margarine, bacon — 3 oz	85	170	20	10	—	—	—	0	20	266	0.5	320	30	0.11	0.22	7.3	—
	Shrimp:																	
157	Canned meat — 3 oz	85	100	21	1	0.1	0.1	Trace	1	98	224	2.6	104	50	0.01	0.03	1.5	—
158	French fried[15] — 3 oz	85	190	17	9	2.3	3.7	2.0	9	61	162	1.7	195	70	0.03	0.07	2.3	—
159	Tuna, canned in oil, drained solids — 3 oz	85	170	24	7	1.7	1.7	0.7	0	7	199	1.6	—	70	0.04	0.10	10.1	—
160	Tuna salad[17] — 1 cup	205	350	30	22	4.3	6.3	6.7	7	41	291	2.7	320	590	0.08	0.23	10.3	2
161	Meat and meat products: Bacon, (20 slices per lb, raw), broiled or fried, crisp — 2 slices	15	85	4	8	2.5	3.7	0.7	Trace	2	34	0.5	35	0	0.08	0.05	0.8	—
	Beef,[18] cooked: Cuts braised, simmered or pot roasted:																	
162	Lean and fat (piece, 2 1/2 by 2 1/2 by 3/4 in) — 3 oz	85	245	23	16	6.8	6.5	0.4	0	10	114	2.9	184	30	0.04	0.18	3.6	—
163	Lean only from item 162 — 2.5 oz	72	140	22	5	2.1	1.8	0.2	0	10	108	2.7	176	10	0.04	0.17	3.3	—
	Ground beef, broiled:																	
164	Lean with 10% fat — 3 oz or patty 3 by 5/8 in	85	185	23	10	4.0	3.9	0.3	0	10	196	3.0	261	20	0.08	0.20	5.1	—
165	Lean with 21% fat — 2.9 oz or patty 3 by 5/8 in	82	235	20	17	7.0	6.7	0.4	0	9	159	2.6	221	30	0.07	0.17	4.4	—
	Roast, oven cooked, no liquid added: Relatively fat, such as rib:																	
166	Lean and fat (2 pieces, 4 1/8 by 2 1/4 by 1/4 in) — 3 oz	85	375	17	33	14.0	13.6	0.8	0	8	158	2.2	189	70	0.05	0.13	3.1	—
	Relatively lean, such as heel of round:																	
167	Lean only from item 166 — 1.8 oz	51	125	14	7	3.0	2.5	0.3	0	6	131	1.8	161	10	0.04	0.11	2.6	—
168	Lean and fat (2 pieces, 4 1/8 by 2 1/4 by 1/4 in) — 3 oz	85	165	25	7	2.8	2.7	0.2	0	11	208	3.2	279	10	0.06	0.19	4.5	—

[13] Based on average vitamin A content of fortified margarine. Federal specifications for fortified margarine require a minimum of 15,000 International Units (I.U.) of vitamin A per pound.
[14] Fatty acid values apply to product made with regular-type margarine.
[15] Dipped in egg, milk or water, and breadcrumbs; fried in vegetable shortening.
[16] If bones are discarded, value for calcium will be greatly reduced.
[17] Dipped in egg, breadcrumbs, and flour or batter.
[18] Prepared with tuna, celery, salad dressing (mayonnaise type), pickle, onion, and egg.
[19] Outer layer of fat on the cut was removed to within approximately 1/2 in of the lean. Deposits of fat within the cut were not removed.

FISH, SHELLFISH, MEAT, POULTRY; RELATED PRODUCTS-Con.

Meat and meat products-Continued
Beef,[15] cooked-Continued
Roast, oven cooked, no liquid added-Continued
Relatively lean such as heel of round-Continued

(A)	(B)	Grams	(C)	(D)	(E)	(F)	(G)	(H)	(I)	(J)	(K)	(L)	(M)	(N)	(O)	(P)	(Q)	(R)	(S)
		Grams	Per cent	Cal- ories	Grams	Grams	Grams	Grams	Grams	Grams	Milli- grams	Milli- grams	Milli- grams	Milli- grams	Inter- national units	Milli- grams	Milli- grams	Milli- grams	Milli- grams
169	Lean only from item 168 --- 2.8 oz	78	65	125	24	3	1.2	1.0	0.1	0	10	199	3.0	268	Trace	0.06	0.18	4.3	—
	Steak. Relatively fat-sirloin, broiled:																		
170	Lean and fat (piece, 2 1/2 by 2 1/2 by 3/4 in) --- 3 oz	85	44	330	20	27	11.3	11.1	.6	0	9	162	2.5	220	50	.05	.15	4.0	—
171	Lean only from item 170 --- 2.0 oz	56	59	115	18	4	1.8	1.6	.2	0	7	146	2.2	202	10	.05	.14	3.6	—
	Relatively lean-round, braised:																		
172	Lean and fat (piece, 4 1/8 by 2 1/4 by 1/2 in) --- 3 oz	85	55	220	24	13	5.5	5.2	.4	0	10	213	3.0	272	20	.07	.19	4.8	—
173	Lean only from item 172 --- 2.4 oz	68	61	130	21	4	1.7	1.5	.2	0	9	182	2.5	238	10	.05	.16	4.1	—
	Beef, canned:																		
174	Corned beef --- 3 oz	85	59	185	22	10	4.9	4.5	.2	0	17	90	3.7	—	—	.01	.20	2.9	0
175	Corned beef hash --- 1 cup	220	67	400	19	25	11.9	10.9	.5	24	29	147	4.4	440	—	.02	.20	2.6	—
176	Beef, dried, chipped --- 2 1/2-oz jar	71	48	145	24	4	2.1	2.0	.1	0	14	287	3.6	142	—	.05	.23	2.7	0
177	Beef and vegetable stew --- 1 cup	245	82	220	16	11	4.9	4.5	.2	15	29	184	2.9	613	2,400	.15	.17	4.7	17
178	Beef potpie (home recipe), baked (piece, 1/3 of 9-in diam. pie) --- 1 piece	210	55	515	21	30	7.9	12.8	6.7	39	29	149	3.8	334	1,720	.30	.30	5.5	6
179	Chili con carne with beans, canned --- 1 cup	255	72	340	19	16	7.5	6.8	.3	31	82	321	4.3	594	150	.08	.18	3.3	—
180	Chop suey with beef and pork (home recipe) --- 1 cup	250	75	300	26	17	8.5	6.2	.7	13	60	248	4.8	425	600	.28	.38	5.0	33
181	Heart, beef, lean, braised --- 3 oz	85	61	160	27	5	1.5	1.1	.6	1	5	154	5.0	197	20	.21	1.04	6.5	1
	Lamb, cooked: Chop, rib (cut 3 per lb with bone), broiled:																		
182	Lean and fat --- 3.1 oz	89	43	360	18	32	14.8	12.1	1.2	0	8	139	1.0	200	—	.11	.19	4.1	—
183	Lean only from item 182 --- 2 oz	57	60	120	16	6	2.5	2.1	.2	0	6	121	1.1	174	—	.09	.15	3.4	—
	Leg, roasted:																		
184	Lean and fat (2 pieces, 4 1/8 by 2 1/4 by 1/4 in) --- 3 oz	85	54	235	22	16	7.3	6.0	.6	0	9	177	1.4	241	—	.13	.23	4.7	—
185	Lean only from item 184 --- 2.5 oz	71	62	130	20	5	2.1	1.8	.2	0	9	169	1.4	227	—	.12	.21	4.4	—
	Shoulder, roasted:																		
186	Lean and fat (3 pieces, 2 1/2 by 2 1/2 by 1/4 in) --- 3 oz	85	50	285	18	23	10.8	8.8	.9	0	9	146	1.0	206	—	.11	.20	4.0	—
187	Lean only from item 186 --- 2.3 oz	64	61	130	17	6	3.6	2.3	.2	0	8	140	1.0	193	—	.10	.18	3.7	—
188	Liver, beef, fried[19] (slice, 6 1/2 by 2 3/8 by 3/8 in) --- 3 oz	85	56	195	22	9	2.5	3.5	.9	5	9	405	7.5	323	[21]45,390	.22	3.56	14.0	23
	Pork, cured, cooked:																		
189	Ham, light cure, lean and fat, roasted (2 pieces, 4 1/8 by 2 1/4 in),[22] --- 3 oz	85	54	245	18	19	6.8	7.9	1.7	0	8	146	2.2	199	0	.40	.15	3.1	—
	Luncheon meat:																		
190	Boiled ham, slice (8 per 8-oz pkg.) --- 1 oz	28	59	65	5	5	1.7	2.0	.4	0	3	47	.8	—	0	.12	.04	.7	—
191	Canned, spiced or unspiced: Slice, approx. 3 by 2 by 1/2 in. --- 1 slice	60	55	175	9	15	5.4	6.7	1.0	1	5	65	1.3	133	0	.19	.13	1.8	—

(A) Item No.	(B) Food, approximate measure, and weight	(C) Water %	(D) Food energy (cal)	(E) Protein (g)	(F) Fat (g)	(G) Saturated (g)	(H) Oleic (g)	(I) Linoleic (g)	(J) Carbohydrate (g)	(K) Calcium (mg)	(L) Phosphorus (mg)	(M) Iron (mg)	(N) Potassium (mg)	(O) Vitamin A (IU)	(P) Thiamin (mg)	(Q) Riboflavin (mg)	(R) Niacin (mg)	(S) Ascorbic acid (mg)
192	Pork, fresh,[18] cooked: Chop, loin (cut 3 per lb with bone), broiled: Lean and fat; 2.7 oz (78 g)	42	305	19	25	8.9	10.4	2.2	0	9	209	2.7	216	0	0.75	0.22	4.5	—
193	Lean only from item 192; 2 oz (56 g)	53	150	17	9	3.1	3.6	.8	0	7	181	2.2	192	0	.63	.18	3.8	—
194	Roast, oven cooked, no liquid added: Lean and fat (piece, 2 1/2 by 2 1/2 by 3/4 in); 3 oz (85 g)	46	310	21	24	8.7	10.2	2.2	0	9	218	2.7	233	0	.78	.22	4.8	—
195	Lean only from item 194; 2.4 oz (68 g)	55	175	20	10	3.5	4.1	.8	0	9	211	2.6	224	0	.73	.21	4.4	—
196	Shoulder cut, simmered: Lean and fat (3 pieces, 2 1/2 by 2 1/2 by 1/4 in); 3 oz (85 g)	46	320	20	26	9.3	10.9	2.3	0	9	118	2.6	158	0	.46	.21	4.1	—
197	Lean only from item 196; 2.2 oz (63 g)	60	135	18	6	2.2	2.6	.6	0	8	111	2.3	146	0	.42	.19	3.7	—
198	Sausages (see also Luncheon Meat (items 190-191)): Bologna, slice (8 per 8-oz pkg.); 1 slice (28 g)	56	85	3	8	3.0	3.4	.5	Trace	2	36	.5	65	—	.05	.06	.7	—
199	Braunschweiger, slice (6 per 6-oz pkg.); 1 slice (28 g)	53	90	4	8	2.6	3.4	.8	1	3	69	1.7	—	1,850	.05	.41	2.3	—
200	Brown and serve (10-11 per 8-oz pkg.), browned; 1 link (17 g)	40	70	3	6	2.3	2.8	.7	Trace	1	—	—	—	—	—	—	—	—
201	Deviled ham, canned; 1 tbsp (13 g)	51	45	2	4	1.5	1.8	.4	0	1	12	.3	—	0	.02	.01	.2	—
202	Frankfurter (8 per 1-lb pkg.), cooked (reheated); 1 frankfurter (56 g)	57	170	7	15	5.6	6.5	1.2	1	3	57	.8	—	—	.08	.11	1.4	—
203	Meat, potted (beef, chicken, turkey), canned; 1 tbsp (13 g)	61	30	2	2	—	—	—	0	1	—	—	35	—	Trace	.03	.2	—
204	Pork link (16 per 1-lb pkg.), cooked; 1 link (13 g)	35	60	2	6	2.1	2.4	.5	Trace	1	21	.3	—	—	.10	.04	.5	—
205	Salami: Dry type, slice (12 per 4-oz pkg.); 1 slice (10 g)	30	45	2	2	1.6	1.6	.1	Trace	1	28	.4	—	—	.04	.03	.5	—
206	Cooked type, slice (8 per 8-oz pkg.); 1 slice (28 g)	51	90	5	7	3.1	3.0	.2	Trace	3	57	.7	—	—	.07	.07	1.2	—
207	Vienna sausage (7 per 4-oz can); 1 sausage (16 g)	63	40	2	3	1.2	1.4	.2	Trace	1	24	.3	—	—	.01	.02	.4	—
208	Veal, medium fat, cooked, bone removed: Cutlet (4 1/8 by 2 1/4 by 1/2 in), braised or broiled; 3 oz (85 g)	60	185	23	9	4.0	3.4	.4	0	9	196	2.7	258	—	.06	.21	4.6	—
209	Rib (2 pieces, 4 1/8 by 2 1/4 by 1/4 in), roasted; 3 oz (85 g)	55	230	23	14	6.1	5.1	.6	0	10	211	2.9	259	—	.11	.26	6.6	—
210	Poultry and poultry products: Chicken, cooked: Breast, fried,[21] bones removed, 1/2 breast (3.3 oz with bones); 2.8 oz (79 g)	58	160	26	5	1.4	1.8	1.1	1	9	218	1.3	—	70	.04	.17	11.6	—
211	Drumstick, fried,[21] bones removed (2 oz with bones); 1.3 oz (38 g)	55	90	12	4	1.1	1.3	.9	Trace	6	89	.9	—	50	.03	.15	2.7	—
212	Half broiler, broiled, bones removed (10.4 oz with bones); 6.2 oz (176 g)	71	240	42	7	2.2	2.5	1.3	0	16	355	3.0	483	160	.09	.34	15.5	—
213	Chicken, canned, boneless; 3 oz (85 g)	65	170	18	10	3.2	3.8	2.0	0	18	210	1.3	117	200	.03	.11	3.7	3
214	Chicken à la king, cooked (home recipe); 1 cup (245 g)	68	470	27	34	12.7	14.3	3.3	12	127	358	2.5	404	1,130	.10	.42	5.4	12
215	Chicken and noodles, cooked (home recipe); 1 cup (240 g)	71	365	22	18	5.9	7.1	3.5	26	26	247	2.2	149	430	.05	.17	4.3	Trace

[18] Outer layer of fat on the cut was removed to within approximately 1/2 in. of the lean. Deposits of fat within the cut were not removed.
[19] Crust made with vegetable shortening and enriched flour.
[20] Regular-type margarine used.
[21] Value varies widely.
[22] About one-fourth of the outer layer of fat on the cut was removed. Deposits of fat within the cut were not removed.
[23] Vegetable shortening used.

FISH, SHELLFISH, MEAT, POULTRY: RELATED PRODUCTS-Con.

(A)	(B)		(C)	(D)	(E)	(F)	(G)	(H)	(I)	(J)	(K)	(L)	(M)	(N)	(O)	(P)	(Q)	(R)	(S)
		Grams	Per cent	Calories	Grams	Grams	Grams	Grams	Grams	Grams	Milligrams	Milligrams	Milligrams	Milligrams	International units	Milligrams	Milligrams	Milligrams	Milligrams
	Poultry and poultry products–Continued																		
	Chicken chow mein:																		
216	Canned---- 1 cup	250	89	95	7	Trace	—	—	—	18	45	35	1.3	418	150	.05	.10	1.0	13
217	From home recipe 1 cup	250	78	255	31	10	2.4	3.4	3.1	10	58	293	2.5	473	280	.08	.23	4.3	10
218	Chicken potpie (home recipe), baked, piece (1/3 or 9-in diam. pie), 1 piece	232	57	545	23	31	11.3	10.9	5.6	42	70	232	3.0	343	3,090	.34	.31	5.5	5
	Turkey, roasted, flesh without skin:																		
219	Dark meat, piece, 2 1/2 by 1 5/8 by 1/4 in, 4 pieces	85	61	175	26	7	2.1	1.5	1.5	0	—	—	2.0	338	—	.03	.20	3.6	—
220	Light meat, piece, 4 by 2 by 1/4 in, 2 pieces	85	62	150	28	3	.9	.6	.7	0	—	—	1.0	349	—	.04	.12	9.4	—
	Light and dark meat:																		
221	Chopped or diced, 1 cup	140	61	265	44	9	2.5	1.7	1.8	0	11	351	2.5	514	—	.07	.25	10.8	—
222	Pieces (1 slice white meat, 4 by 2 by 1/4 in with 2 slices dark meat, 2 1/2 by 1 5/8 by 1/4 in), 3 pieces	85	61	160	27	5	1.5	1.0	1.1	0	7	213	1.5	312	—	.04	.15	6.5	—

FRUITS AND FRUIT PRODUCTS

(A)	(B)		(C)	(D)	(E)	(F)	(G)	(H)	(I)	(J)	(K)	(L)	(M)	(N)	(O)	(P)	(Q)	(R)	(S)
	Apples, raw, unpeeled, without cores:																		
223	2 3/4-in diam. (about 3 per lb with cores), 1 apple	138	84	80	Trace	Trace	—	—	—	20	10	14	.4	152	120	.04	.03	.1	6
224	3 1/4-in diam. (about 2 per lb with cores), 1 apple	212	84	125	Trace	1	—	—	—	31	15	21	.6	233	190	.06	.04	.2	8
225	Applejuice, bottled or canned, 1 cup	248	88	120	Trace	Trace	—	—	—	30	15	22	1.5	250	—	.02	.05	.2	[12]2
	Applesauce, canned:																		
226	Sweetened, 1 cup	255	76	230	1	Trace	—	—	—	61	10	13	1.3	166	100	.05	.03	.1	[13]3
227	Unsweetened, 1 cup	244	89	100	Trace	Trace	—	—	—	26	10	12	1.2	190	100	.05	.02	.1	[12]2
	Apricots:																		
228	Raw, without pits (about 12 per lb with pits), 3 apricots	107	85	55	1	Trace	—	—	—	14	18	25	.5	301	2,890	.03	.04	.6	11
229	Canned in heavy syrup (halves and syrup), 1 cup	258	77	220	2	Trace	—	—	—	57	28	39	.8	604	4,490	.05	.05	1.0	10
	Dried:																		
230	Uncooked (28 large or 37 medium halves per cup), 1 cup	130	25	340	7	1	—	—	—	86	87	140	7.2	1,273	14,170	.01	.21	4.3	16
231	Cooked, unsweetened, Fruit and liquid, 1 cup	250	76	215	4	1	—	—	—	54	55	88	4.5	795	7,500	.01	.13	2.5	8
232	Apricot nectar, canned, 1 cup	251	85	145	1	Trace	—	—	—	37	23	30	.5	379	2,380	.03	.03	.5	[24]36
	Avocados, raw, whole, without skins and seeds:																		
233	California, mid- and late-winter (with skin and seed, 3 1/8-in diam.; wt. 10 oz), 1 avocado	216	74	370	5	37	5.5	22.0	3.7	13	22	91	1.3	1,303	630	.24	.43	3.5	30
234	Florida, late summer and fall (with skin and seed, 3 5/8-in diam.; wt. 1 lb), 1 avocado	304	78	390	4	33	6.7	15.7	5.3	27	30	128	1.8	1,836	880	.33	.61	4.9	43
235	Banana without peel (about 2.6 per lb with peel), 1 banana	119	76	100	1	Trace	—	—	—	26	10	31	.8	440	230	.06	.07	.8	12
236	Banana flakes, 1 tbsp	6	3	20	Trace	Trace	—	—	—	5	2	6	.2	92	50	.01	.01	.2	Trace

(A)	(B)	(g)	(C)	(D)	(E)	(F)	(G)	(H)	(I)	(J)	(K)	(L)	(M)	(N)	(O)	(P)	(Q)	(R)	(S)
237	Blackberries, raw --------- 1 cup	144	85	85	2	1	—	—	—	19	46	27	1.3	245	290	0.04	0.06	0.6	30
238	Blueberries, raw --------- 1 cup	145	83	90	2	1	—	—	—	22	22	19	1.5	117	150	.04	.09	.7	20
	Cantaloup. See Muskmelons (item 271).																		
	Cherries:																			
239	Sour (tart), red, pitted, canned, water pack --- 1 cup	244	88	105	2	Trace	—	—	—	26	37	32	.7	317	1,660	.07	.05	.5	12
240	Sweet, raw, without pits and stems --- 10 cherries	68	80	45	1	Trace	—	—	—	12	15	13	.3	129	70	.03	.04	.3	7
241	Cranberry juice cocktail, bottled, sweetened --- 1 cup	253	83	165	Trace	Trace	—	—	—	42	13	8	.8	25	Trace	.03	.03	.1	[26]81
242	Cranberry sauce, sweetened, canned, strained --- 1 cup	277	62	405	Trace	1	—	—	—	104	17	11	.6	83	60	.03	.03	.1	6
	Dates:																			
243	Whole, without pits --- 10 dates	80	23	220	2	Trace	—	—	—	58	47	50	2.4	518	40	.07	.08	1.8	0
244	Chopped --- 1 cup	178	23	490	4	1	—	—	—	130	105	112	5.3	1,153	90	.16	.18	3.9	0
245	Fruit cocktail, canned, in heavy sirup --- 1 cup	255	80	195	1	Trace	—	—	—	50	23	31	1.0	411	360	.05	.03	1.0	5
	Grapefruit:																			
	Raw, medium, 3 3/4-in diam. (about 1 lb 1 oz):																			
246	Pink or red --- 1/2 grapefruit with peel[30]	241	89	50	1	Trace	—	—	—	13	20	20	.5	166	540	.05	.02	.2	44
247	White --- 1/2 grapefruit with peel[30]	241	89	45	1	Trace	—	—	—	12	19	19	.5	159	10	.05	.02	.2	44
248	Canned, sections with sirup --- 1 cup	254	81	180	2	Trace	—	—	—	45	33	36	.8	343	30	.08	.05	.5	76
	Grapefruit juice:																			
249	Raw, pink, red, or white --- 1 cup	246	90	95	1	Trace	—	—	—	23	22	37	.5	399	(31)	.10	.05	.5	93
	Canned, white:																			
250	Unsweetened --- 1 cup	247	89	100	1	Trace	—	—	—	24	20	35	1.0	400	20	.07	.05	.5	84
251	Sweetened --- 1 cup	250	86	135	1	Trace	—	—	—	32	20	35	1.0	405	30	.08	.05	.5	78
	Frozen concentrate, unsweetened:																			
252	Undiluted, 6-fl oz can --- 1 can	207	62	300	4	1	—	—	—	72	70	124	.8	1,250	60	.29	.12	1.4	286
253	Diluted with 3 parts water by volume --- 1 cup	247	89	100	1	Trace	—	—	—	24	25	42	.2	420	20	.10	.04	.5	96
254	Dehydrated crystals, prepared with water (1 lb yields about 1 gal) --- 1 cup	247	90	100	1	Trace	—	—	—	24	22	40	.2	412	20	.10	.05	.5	91
	Grapes, European type (adherent skin), raw:																			
255	Thompson Seedless --- 10 grapes	50	81	35	Trace	Trace	—	—	—	9	6	10	.2	87	50	.03	.02	.2	2
256	Tokay and Emperor, seeded types --- 10 grapes[32]	60	81	40	Trace	Trace	—	—	—	10	7	11	.2	99	60	.03	.02	.2	2
	Grapejuice:																			
257	Canned or bottled --- 1 cup	253	83	165	1	Trace	—	—	—	42	28	30	.8	293	—	.10	.05	.5	[26]Trace
	Frozen concentrate, sweetened:																			
258	Undiluted, 6-fl oz can --- 1 can	216	53	395	1	Trace	—	—	—	100	22	32	.9	255	40	.13	.22	1.5	[32]32
259	Diluted with 3 parts water by volume --- 1 cup	250	86	135	1	Trace	—	—	—	33	8	10	.3	85	10	.05	.08	.5	[32]10
260	Grape drink, canned --- 1 cup	250	86	135	Trace	Trace	—	—	—	35	8	10	.3	88	[32]10	.03	.03	.3	(32)
261	Lemon, raw, size 165, without peel and seeds (about 4 per lb with peels and seeds) --- 1 lemon[33]	74	90	20	1	Trace	—	—	—	6	19	12	.4	102	10	.03	.01	.1	39
	Lemon juice:																			
262	Raw --- 1 cup	244	91	60	1	Trace	—	—	—	20	17	24	.5	344	50	.07	.02	.2	112
263	Canned, or bottled, unsweetened --- 1 cup	244	92	55	1	Trace	—	—	—	19	13	24	.5	344	50	.07	.02	.2	102
264	Frozen, single strength, unsweetened, 6-fl oz can --- 1 can	183	92	40	1	Trace	—	—	—	13	13	16	.5	258	40	.05	.02	.2	81
	Lemonade concentrate, frozen:																			
265	Undiluted, 6-fl oz can --- 1 can	219	49	425	Trace	Trace	—	—	—	112	9	13	.4	153	40	.07	.06	.7	66
266	Diluted with 4 1/3 parts water by volume --- 1 cup	248	89	105	Trace	Trace	—	—	—	28	2	3	.1	40	10	.01	.02	.2	17

[1]Crust made with vegetable shortening and enriched flour.

[26]Also applies to pasteurized apple cider.

[27]Applies to product without added ascorbic acid. For value of product with added ascorbic acid, refer to label.

[28]Based on product with label claim of 45% of U.S. RDA in 6 fl oz.

[29]Based on product with label claim of 100% of U.S. RDA in 6 fl oz.

[30]Weight includes peel and membranes between sections. Without these parts, the weight of the edible portion is 123 g for item 246 and 118 g for item 247.

[31]For white-fleshed varieties, value is about 20 International Units (I.U.) per cup; for red-fleshed varieties, 1,080 I.U.

[32]Weight includes seeds. Without seeds, weight of the edible portion is 57 g.

[33]Weight includes peel. Without peel, the weight of the edible portion is 57 g.

[32]Based on claim that 6 fl oz of reconstituted juice contain 45% or 50% of the U.S. RDA, value in milligrams is 108 or 120 for a 6-fl oz can (item 256), 36 or 40 for 1 cup of diluted juice (item 259).

[33]For products with added thiamin and riboflavin but without added ascorbic acid, values in milligrams would be 0.60 for thiamin, 0.80 for riboflavin, and trace for ascorbic acid. For products with only ascorbic acid added, value varies with the brand. Consult the label.

(A)	(B)		(C) Per cent	(D) Cal-ories	(E) Grams	(F) Grams	(G) Grams	(H) Grams	(I) Grams	(J) Grams	(K) Milli-grams	(L) Milli-grams	(M) Milli-grams	(N) Milli-grams	(O) Inter-national units	(P) Milli-grams	(Q) Milli-grams	(R) Milli-grams	(S) Milli-grams
	FRUITS AND FRUIT PRODUCTS-Con.	Grams																	
	Limeade concentrate, frozen:																		
267	Undiluted, 6-fl oz can --- 1 can	218	50	410	Trace	Trace	---	---	---	108	11	13	0.2	129	Trace	0.02	0.02	0.2	26
268	Diluted with 4 1/3 parts water by volume. --- 1 cup	247	89	100	Trace	Trace	---	---	---	27	3	3	Trace	32	Trace	Trace	Trace	Trace	6
	Limejuice:																		
269	Raw --- 1 cup	246	90	65	1	Trace	---	---	---	22	22	27	.5	256	20	.05	.02	.2	79
270	Canned, unsweetened --- 1 cup	246	90	65	1	Trace	---	---	---	22	22	27	.5	256	20	.05	.02	.2	52
	Muskmelons, raw, with rind, without seed cavity:																		
271	Cantaloup, orange-fleshed (with rind and seed cavity, 5-in diam., 2 1/3 lb). --- 1/2 melon with rind[33]	477	91	80	2	Trace	---	---	---	20	38	44	1.1	682	9,240	.11	.08	1.6	90
272	Honeydew (with rind and seed cavity, 6 1/2-in diam., 5 1/4 lb). --- 1/10 melon with rind[33]	226	91	50	1	Trace	---	---	---	11	21	24	.6	374	60	.06	.04	.9	34
	Oranges, all commercial varieties:																		
273	Whole, 2 5/8-in diam., without peel and seeds (about 2 1/2 per lb with peel and seeds). --- 1 orange	131	86	65	1	Trace	---	---	---	16	54	26	.5	263	260	.13	.05	.5	66
274	Sections without membranes --- 1 cup	180	86	90	2	Trace	---	---	---	22	74	36	.7	360	360	.18	.07	.7	90
	Orange juice:																		
275	Raw, all varieties --- 1 cup	248	88	110	2	Trace	---	---	---	26	27	42	.5	496	500	.22	.07	1.0	124
276	Canned, unsweetened --- 1 cup	249	87	120	2	Trace	---	---	---	28	25	45	1.0	496	500	.17	.05	.7	100
	Frozen concentrate:																		
277	Undiluted, 6-fl oz can --- 1 can	213	55	360	5	Trace	---	---	---	87	75	126	.9	1,500	1,620	.68	.11	2.8	360
278	Diluted with 3 parts water by volume. --- 1 cup	249	87	120	2	Trace	---	---	---	29	25	42	.2	503	540	.23	.03	.9	120
279	Dehydrated crystals, prepared with water (1 lb yields about 1 gal). --- 1 cup	248	88	115	1	Trace	---	---	---	27	25	40	.5	518	500	.20	.07	1.0	109
	Orange and grapefruit juice:																		
	Frozen concentrate:																		
280	Undiluted, 6-fl oz can --- 1 can	210	59	330	4	1	---	---	---	78	61	99	.8	1,308	800	.48	.06	2.3	302
281	Diluted with 3 parts water by volume. --- 1 cup	248	88	110	1	Trace	---	---	---	26	20	32	.2	439	270	.15	.02	.7	102
282	Papayas, raw, 1/2-in cubes --- 1 cup	140	89	55	1	Trace	---	---	---	14	28	22	.4	328	2,450	.06	.06	.4	78
	Peaches:																		
	Raw:																		
283	Whole, 2 1/2-in diam., peeled, pitted (about 4 per lb with peels and pits). --- 1 peach	100	89	40	1	Trace	---	---	---	10	9	19	.5	202	[33]1,330	.02	.05	1.0	7
284	Sliced --- 1 cup	170	89	65	1	Trace	---	---	---	16	15	32	.9	343	[32]2,260	.03	.09	1.7	12
	Canned, yellow-fleshed, solids and liquid (halves or slices):																		
285	Sirup pack --- 1 cup	256	79	200	1	Trace	---	---	---	51	10	31	.8	333	1,100	.03	.05	1.5	8
286	Water pack --- 1 cup	244	91	75	1	Trace	---	---	---	20	10	32	.7	334	1,100	.02	.07	1.5	7
	Dried:																		
287	Uncooked --- 1 cup	160	25	420	5	1	---	---	---	109	77	187	9.6	1,520	6,240	.02	.30	8.5	29
288	Cooked, unsweetened, halves and juice. --- 1 cup	250	77	205	3	1	---	---	---	54	38	93	4.8	743	3,050	.01	.15	3.8	5

(A)	(B)	(grams)	(C)	(D)	(E)	(F)	(G)	(H)	(I)	(J)	(K)	(L)	(M)	(N)	(O)	(P)	(Q)	(R)	(S)
289	Frozen, sliced, sweetened: 1 container	284	77	250	1	Trace	—	—	—	64	10	37	1.4	352	1,850	0.03	0.11	2.0	[34]116
290	1 cup	250	77	220	1	Trace	—	—	—	57	10	33	1.3	310	1,630	.03	.10	1.8	[34]103
291	Pears: Raw, with skin, cored: Bartlett, 2 1/2-in diam. (about 2 1/2 per lb with cores and stems) — 1 pear	164	83	100	1	1	—	—	—	25	13	18	.5	213	30	.03	.07	.2	7
292	Bosc, 2 1/2-in diam. (about 3 per lb with cores and stems) — 1 pear	141	83	85	1	1	—	—	—	22	11	16	.4	83	30	.03	.06	.1	6
293	D'Anjou, 3-in diam. (about 2 per lb with cores and stems) — 1 pear	200	83	120	1	1	—	—	—	31	16	22	.6	260	40	.04	.08	.2	8
294	Canned, solids and liquid, sirup pack, heavy (halves or slices) — 1 cup	255	80	195	1	1	—	—	—	50	13	18	.5	214	10	.03	.05	.3	3
295	Pineapple: Raw, diced — 1 cup	155	85	80	1	Trace	—	—	—	21	26	12	.8	226	110	.14	.05	.3	26
296	Canned, heavy sirup pack, solids and liquid: Crushed, chunks, tidbits — 1 cup	255	80	190	1	Trace	—	—	—	49	28	13	.8	245	130	.20	.05	.3	18
297	Slices and liquid: Large — 1 slice; 2 1/4 tbsp liquid	105	80	80	Trace	Trace	—	—	—	20	12	5	.3	101	50	.08	.02	.2	7
298	Medium — 1 slice; 1 1/4 tbsp liquid	58	80	45	Trace	Trace	—	—	—	11	6	3	.2	56	30	.05	.01	.1	4
299	Pineapple juice, unsweetened, canned — 1 cup	250	86	140	1	Trace	—	—	—	34	38	23	.8	373	130	.13	.05	.5	[26]80
300	Plums: Raw, without pits: Japanese and hybrid (2 1/8-in diam., about 6 1/2 per lb with pits) — 1 plum	66	87	30	Trace	Trace	—	—	—	8	8	12	.3	112	160	.02	.02	.3	4
301	Prune-type (1 1/2-in diam., about 15 per lb with pits) — 1 plum	28	79	20	Trace	Trace	—	—	—	6	3	5	.1	48	80	.01	.01	.1	1
302	Canned, heavy sirup pack (Italian prunes), with pits and liquid: 1 cup[35]	272	77	215	1	Trace	—	—	—	56	23	26	2.3	367	3,130	.05	.05	1.0	5
303	3 plums; 2 3/4 tbsp liquid[35]	140	77	110	1	Trace	—	—	—	29	12	13	1.2	189	1,610	.03	.03	.5	3
304	Prunes, dried, "softenized," with pits: Uncooked — 4 extra large or 5 large prunes[35]	49	28	110	1	Trace	—	—	—	29	22	34	1.7	298	690	.04	.07	.7	1
305	Cooked, unsweetened, all sizes, fruit and liquid — 1 cup[35]	250	66	255	2	1	—	—	—	67	51	79	3.8	695	1,590	.07	.15	1.5	2
306	Prune juice, canned or bottled — 1 cup	256	80	195	1	Trace	—	—	—	49	36	51	1.8	602	—	.03	.03	1.0	5
307	Raisins, seedless: Cup, not pressed down — 1 cup	145	18	420	4	Trace	—	—	—	112	90	146	5.1	1,106	30	.16	.12	.7	1
308	Packet, 1/2 oz (1 1/2 tbsp) — 1 packet	14	18	40	Trace	Trace	—	—	—	11	9	14	.5	107	Trace	.02	.01	.1	Trace
309	Raspberries, red: Raw, capped, whole — 1 cup	123	84	70	1	1	—	—	—	17	27	27	1.1	207	160	.04	.11	1.1	31
310	Frozen, sweetened, 10-oz container — 1 container	284	74	280	2	1	—	—	—	70	37	48	1.7	284	200	.06	.17	1.7	60
311	Rhubarb, cooked, added sugar: From raw — 1 cup	270	63	380	1	Trace	—	—	—	97	211	41	1.6	548	220	.05	.14	.7	16
312	From frozen, sweetened — 1 cup	270	63	385	1	1	—	—	—	98	211	32	1.9	475	190	.05	.11	.5	16

[26] Based on product with label claim of 100% of U.S. RDA in 6 fl oz.

[27] Weight includes rind. Without rind, the weight of the edible portion is 272 g for item 271 and 149 g for item 272.

[33] Represents yellow-fleshed varieties. For white-fleshed varieties, value is 50 International Units (I.U.) for 1 peach, 90 I.U. for 1 cup of slices.

[34] Value represents products without added ascorbic acid. For products with added ascorbic acid, value in milligrams is 116 for a 10-oz container, 103 for 1 cup.

[35] Weight includes pits. After removal of the pits, the weight of the edible portion is 258 g for item 302, 133 g for item 303, 43 g for item 304, and 213 g for item 305.

(A)	(B)		Grams	(C) Per-cent	(D) Cal-ories	(E) Grams	(F) Grams	(G) Grams	(H) Grams	(I) Grams	(J) Grams	(K) Milli-grams	(L) Milli-grams	(M) Milli-grams	(N) Milli-grams	(O) Inter-national units	(P) Milli-grams	(Q) Milli-grams	(R) Milli-grams	(S) Milli-grams
	FRUITS AND FRUIT PRODUCTS—Con.																			
313	Strawberries: Raw, whole berries, capped	1 cup	149	90	55	1	1	—	—	—	13	31	31	1.5	244	90	0.04	0.10	0.9	88
	Frozen, sweetened:																			
314	Sliced, 10-oz container	1 container	284	71	310	1	1	—	—	—	79	40	48	2.0	318	90	.06	.17	1.4	151
315	Whole, 1-lb container (about 1 3/4 cups)	1 container	454	76	415	2	1	—	—	—	107	59	73	2.7	472	140	.09	.27	2.3	249
316	Tangerine, raw, 2 3/8-in diam., size 176, without peel (about 4 per lb with peels and seeds)	1 tangerine	86	87	40	1	Trace	—	—	—	10	34	15	.3	108	360	.05	.02	.1	27
317	Tangerine juice, canned, sweetened	1 cup	249	87	125	1	Trace	—	—	—	30	44	35	.5	440	1,040	.15	.05	.2	54
318	Watermelon, raw, 4 by 8 in wedge with rind and seeds (1/16 of 32 2/3-lb melon, 10 by 16 in)	1 wedge with rind and seeds[17]	926	93	110	2	1	—	—	—	27	30	43	2.1	426	2,510	.13	.13	.9	30
	GRAIN PRODUCTS																			
319	Bagel, 3-in diam.: Egg	1 bagel	55	32	165	6	2	0.5	0.9	0.8	28	9	43	1.2	41	30	.14	.10	1.2	0
320	Water	1 bagel	55	29	165	6	2	.2	.4	.6	30	8	41	1.2	42	0	.15	.11	1.4	0
321	Barley, pearled, light, uncooked	1 cup	200	11	700	16	2	.3	.2	.8	158	32	378	4.0	320	0	.24	.10	6.2	0
	Biscuits, baking powder, 2-in diam. (enriched flour, vegetable shortening):																			
322	From home recipe	1 biscuit	28	27	105	2	5	1.2	2.0	1.2	13	34	49	.4	33	Trace	.08	.08	.7	Trace
323	From mix	1 biscuit	28	29	90	2	3	.6	1.1	.7	15	19	65	.6	32	Trace	.09	.08	.8	Trace
324	Breadcrumbs (enriched):[18] Dry, grated	1 cup	100	7	390	13	5	1.0	1.6	1.4	73	122	141	3.6	152	Trace	.35	.35	4.8	Trace
	Breads: See white bread (items 349-350).																			
325	Boston brown bread, canned, slice 3 1/4 by 1/2 in.[18]	1 slice	45	45	95	2	1	.1	.2	.2	21	41	72	.9	131	[19]0	.06	.04	.7	0
	Cracked-wheat bread (3/4 enriched wheat flour, 1/4 cracked wheat):[18]																			
326	Loaf, 1 lb	1 loaf	454	35	1,195	39	10	2.2	3.0	3.9	236	399	581	9.5	608	Trace	1.52	1.13	14.4	Trace
327	Slice (18 per loaf)	1 slice	25	35	65	2	1	.1	.2	.2	13	22	32	.5	34	Trace	.08	.06	.8	Trace
	French or vienna bread, enriched:[18]																			
328	Loaf, 1 lb	1 loaf	454	31	1,315	41	14	3.2	4.7	4.6	251	195	386	10.0	408	Trace	1.80	1.10	15.0	Trace
	Slice:																			
329	French (5 by 2 1/2 by 1 in)	1 slice	35	31	100	3	1	.2	.4	.4	19	15	30	.8	32	Trace	.14	.08	1.2	Trace
330	Vienna (4 3/4 by 4 by 1/2 in)	1 slice	25	31	75	2	1	.2	.3	.3	14	11	21	.6	23	Trace	.10	.06	.8	Trace
	Italian bread, enriched:																			
331	Loaf, 1 lb	1 loaf	454	32	1,250	41	4	.6	Trace	1.5	256	77	349	10.0	336	0	1.80	1.10	15.0	0
332	Slice, 4 1/2 by 3 1/4 by 3/4 in	1 slice	30	32	85	3	Trace	Trace	Trace	.1	17	5	23	.7	22	0	.12	.07	1.0	0
	Raisin bread, enriched:[18]																			
333	Loaf, 1 lb	1 loaf	454	35	1,190	30	13	3.0	4.7	3.9	243	322	395	10.0	1,057	Trace	1.70	1.07	10.7	Trace
334	Slice (18 per loaf)	1 slice	25	35	65	2	1	.2	.3	.2	13	18	22	.6	58	Trace	.09	.06	.6	Trace

(A) No.	(B) Food, approximate measure	Grams	(C) Water %	(D) Food energy	(E) Protein (g)	(F) Fat (g)	(G) Sat.	(H) Oleic	(I) Linoleic	(J) Carbo.	(K) Ca (mg)	(L) P (mg)	(M) Fe (mg)	(N) K (mg)	(O) Vit. A	(P) Thiamin	(Q) Ribo.	(R) Niacin	(S) Asc.
	Rye Bread:																		
	American, light (2/3 enriched wheat flour, 1/3 rye flour):																		
335	Loaf, 1 lb — 1 loaf	454	36	1,100	41	5	0.7	0.5	2.2	236	340	667	9.1	658	0	1.35	0.98	12.9	0
336	Slice (4¾ by 3¾ by 7/16 in) — 1 slice	25	36	60	2	Trace	Trace	Trace	.1	13	19	37	.5	36	0	.07	.05	.7	0
	Pumpernickel (2/3 rye flour, 1/3 enriched wheat flour):																		
337	Loaf, 1 lb — 1 loaf	454	34	1,115	41	5	.7	.5	2.4	241	381	1,039	11.8	2,059	0	1.30	.93	8.5	0
338	Slice (5 by 4 by 3/8 in) — 1 slice	32	34	80	3	Trace	.1	Trace	.2	17	27	73	.8	145	0	.09	.07	.6	0
	White bread, enriched:[18]																		
	Soft-crumb type:																		
339	Loaf, 1 lb — 1 loaf	454	36	1,225	39	15	3.4	5.3	4.6	229	381	440	11.3	476	Trace	1.80	1.10	15.0	Trace
340	Slice (18 per loaf) — 1 slice	25	36	70	2	1	.2	.3	.3	13	21	24	.6	26	Trace	.10	.06	.8	Trace
341	Slice, toasted — 1 slice	22	25	70	2	1	.2	.3	.2	13	21	24	.6	26	Trace	.08	.06	.8	Trace
342	Slice (22 per loaf) — 1 slice	20	36	55	2	1	.2	.2	.2	10	17	19	.5	21	Trace	.08	.05	.7	Trace
343	Slice, toasted — 1 slice	17	25	55	2	1	.2	.2	.2	10	17	19	.5	21	Trace	.06	.05	.7	Trace
344	Loaf, 1½ lb — 1 loaf	680	36	1,835	59	22	5.2	7.9	6.9	343	571	660	17.0	714	Trace	2.70	1.65	22.5	Trace
345	Slice (24 per loaf) — 1 slice	28	36	75	2	1	.2	.3	.3	14	24	27	.7	29	Trace	.11	.07	.9	Trace
346	Slice, toasted — 1 slice	24	25	75	2	1	.2	.3	.3	14	24	27	.7	25	Trace	.09	.07	.9	Trace
347	Slice (28 per loaf) — 1 slice	24	36	65	2	1	.2	.3	.2	12	20	23	.6	25	Trace	.10	.06	.8	Trace
348	Slice, toasted — 1 slice	21	25	65	2	1	.2	.3	.2	12	20	23	.6	25	Trace	.08	.06	.8	Trace
349	Cubes — 1 cup	30	36	80	3	1	.2	.3	.3	15	25	25	.7	32	Trace	.12	.07	1.0	Trace
350	Crumbs — 1 cup	45	36	120	4	2	.3	.5	.5	23	38	44	1.1	47	Trace	.18	.11	1.5	Trace
	Firm-crumb type:																		
351	Loaf, 1 lb — 1 loaf	454	35	1,245	41	17	3.9	5.9	5.2	228	435	463	11.3	549	Trace	1.80	1.10	15.0	Trace
352	Slice (20 per loaf) — 1 slice	23	35	65	2	1	.2	.3	.3	12	22	23	.6	28	Trace	.09	.06	.8	Trace
353	Slice, toasted — 1 slice	20	24	65	2	1	.2	.3	.3	12	22	23	.6	28	Trace	.07	.06	.8	Trace
354	Loaf, 2 lb — 1 loaf	907	35	2,495	82	34	7.7	11.8	10.4	455	871	925	22.7	1,097	Trace	3.60	2.20	30.0	Trace
355	Slice (34 per loaf) — 1 slice	27	35	75	2	1	.2	.3	.3	14	26	28	.7	33	Trace	.11	.06	.9	Trace
356	Slice, toasted — 1 slice	23	24	75	2	1	.2	.3	.3	14	26	28	.7	33	Trace	.09	.06	.9	Trace
	Whole-wheat bread:																		
	Soft-crumb type:[18]																		
357	Loaf, 1 lb — 1 loaf	454	36	1,095	41	12	2.2	2.9	4.2	224	449	1,152	13.6	1,161	Trace	1.37	.45	12.7	Trace
358	Slice (16 per loaf) — 1 slice	28	36	65	3	1	.1	.2	.2	14	25	71	.8	72	Trace	.09	.03	.8	Trace
359	Slice, toasted — 1 slice	24	24	65	3	1	.1	.2	.2	14	25	71	.8	72	Trace	.07	.03	.8	Trace
	Firm-crumb type:[18]																		
360	Loaf, 1 lb — 1 loaf	454	36	1,100	48	14	2.5	3.3	4.9	216	381	1,034	13.6	1,238	Trace	1.17	.54	12.7	Trace
361	Slice (18 per loaf) — 1 slice	25	36	60	3	1	.1	.2	.3	12	24	57	.8	68	Trace	.06	.03	.7	Trace
362	Slice, toasted — 1 slice	21	24	60	3	1	.1	.2	.3	12	24	57	.8	68	Trace	.05	.03	.7	Trace
	Breakfast cereals:																		
	Hot type, cooked:																		
	Corn (hominy) grits, degermed:																		
363	Enriched — 1 cup	245	87	125	3	Trace	Trace	Trace	Trace	27	2	25	.7	27	Trace[19]	.10	.07	1.0	0
364	Unenriched — 1 cup	245	87	125	3	Trace	Trace	Trace	Trace	27	2	25	.2	27	Trace[19]	.05	.02	.5	0
365	Farina, quick-cooking, enriched — 1 cup	245	89	105	3	Trace	Trace	Trace	Trace	22	147	113[45]	[44]	25	0	.12	.07	1.0	0
366	Oatmeal or rolled oats — 1 cup	240	87	130	5	2	.4	.8	.9	23	22	137	1.4	146	0	.19	.05	.2	0
367	Wheat, rolled — 1 cup	240	80	180	5	1	—	—	—	41	19	182	1.7	202	0	.17	.07	2.2	0
368	Wheat, whole-meal — 1 cup	245	88	110	4	1	—	—	—	23	17	127	1.2	118	0	.15	.05	1.5	0
	Ready-to-eat:																		
369	Bran flakes (40% bran), added sugar, salt, iron, vitamins — 1 cup	35	3	105	4	1	—	—	—	28	19	125	15.6	137	1,650	.41	.49	4.1	12
370	Bran flakes with raisins, added sugar, salt, iron, vitamins — 1 cup	50	7	145	4	1	—	—	—	40	28	146	16.9	154	2,350	.58	.71	5.8	18

[17] Weight includes rind and seeds. Without rind and seeds, weight of the edible portion is 426 g.

[18] Made with vegetable shortening.

[19] Applies to product made with white cornmeal. With yellow cornmeal, value is 30 International Units (I.U.).

[44] Applies to white varieties. For yellow varieties, value is 150 International Units (I.U.).

[45] Applies to products that do not contain di-sodium phosphate. If di-sodium phosphate is an ingredient, value is 162 mg.

[46] Value may range from less than 1 mg to about 8 mg depending on the brand. Consult the label.

(A)	(B) GRAIN PRODUCTS—Con.	Grams	(C) Per cent	(D) Cal-ories	(E) Grams	(F) Grams	(G) Grams	(H) Grams	(I) Grams	(J) Grams	(K) Milli-grams	(L) Milli-grams	(M) Milli-grams	(N) Milli-grams	(O) Inter-national units	(P) Milli-grams	(Q) Milli-grams	(R) Milli-grams	(S) Milli-grams
	Breakfast cereals—Continued																		
	Ready-to-eat—Continued																		
	Corn flakes:																		
371	Plain, added sugar, salt, iron, vitamins. 1 cup	25	4	95	2	Trace	—	—	—	21	(*)	9	0.6	30	1,180	0.29	0.35	2.9	9
372	Sugar-coated, added salt, iron, vitamins. 1 cup	40	2	155	2	Trace	—	—	—	37	1	10	1.0	27	1,880	.46	.56	4.6	14
373	Corn, puffed, plain, added sugar, salt, iron, vita-mins. 1 cup	20	4	80	2	1	—	—	—	16	4	18	2.3	—	940	.23	.28	2.3	7
374	Corn, shredded, added sugar, salt, iron, thiamin, niacin. 1 cup	25	3	95	2	Trace	—	—	—	22	1	10	.6	—	0	.11	.05	.5	0
375	Oats, puffed, added sugar, salt, minerals, vitamins. 1 cup	25	3	100	3	1	—	—	—	19	44	102	2.9	—	1,180	.29	.35	2.9	9
376	Rice, puffed: Plain, added iron, thiamin, niacin. 1 cup	15	4	60	1	Trace	—	—	—	13	3	14	.3	15	0	.07	.01	.7	0
377	Presweetened, added salt, iron, vitamins. 1 cup	28	3	115	1	0	—	—	—	26	3	14	**1.1	43	1,250	.38	.43	5.0	*15
378	Wheat flakes, added sugar, salt, iron, vitamins. 1 cup	30	4	105	3	Trace	—	—	—	24	12	83	(**)	81	1,410	.35	.42	3.5	11
	Wheat, puffed:																		
379	Plain, added iron, thiamin, niacin. 1 cup	15	3	55	2	Trace	—	—	—	12	4	48	.6	51	0	.08	.03	1.2	0
380	Presweetened, added salt, iron, vitamins. 1 cup	38	3	140	3	Trace	—	—	—	33	7	52	**1.6	63	1,680	.50	.57	6.7	*20
381	Wheat, shredded, plain. 1 oblong biscuit or 1/2 cup spoon-size biscuits.	25	7	90	2	1	—	—	—	20	11	97	.9	87	0	.06	.03	1.1	0
382	Wheat germ, without salt and sugar, toasted. 1 tbsp.	6	4	25	2	1	—	—	—	3	3	70	.5	57	10	.11	.05	.3	1
383	Buckwheat flour, light, sifted. 1 cup	98	12	340	6	1	0.2	0.4	0.4	78	11	86	1.0	314	0	.08	.04	.4	0
384	Bulgur, canned, seasoned. 1 cup	135	56	245	8	4	—	—	—	44	27	263	1.9	151	0	.08	.05	4.1	0
	Cake icings. See Sugars and Sweets (items 532-536).																		
	Cakes made from cake mixes with enriched flour:[4]																		
	Angelfood:																		
385	Whole cake (9 3/4-in diam. tube cake). 1 cake	635	34	1,645	36	1	—	—	—	377	603	756	2.5	381	0	.37	.95	3.6	0
386	Piece, 1/12 of cake. 1 piece	53	34	135	3	Trace	—	—	—	32	50	63	.2	32	0	.03	.08	.3	0
	Coffeecake:																		
387	Whole cake (7 3/4 by 5 5/8 by 1 1/4 in). 1 cake	430	30	1,385	27	41	11.7	16.3	8.8	225	262	748	6.9	469	690	.82	.91	7.7	0
388	Piece, 1/6 of cake. 1 piece	72	30	230	5	7	2.0	2.7	1.5	38	44	125	1.2	78	120	.14	.15	1.3	Trace
	Cupcakes, made with egg, milk, 2 1/2-in diam.:																		
389	Without icing. 1 cupcake	25	26	90	1	3	.8	1.2	.7	14	40	59	.3	21	40	.05	.05	.4	Trace
390	With chocolate icing. 1 cupcake	36	22	130	2	5	2.0	1.6	.6	21	47	71	.4	42	60	.05	.06	.4	Trace
	Devil's food with chocolate icing:																		
391	Whole, 2 layer cake (8- or 9-in diam.). 1 cake	1,107	24	3,755	49	136	50.0	44.9	17.0	645	653	1,162	16.6	1,439	1,660	1.06	1.65	10.1	1
392	Piece, 1/16 of cake. 1 piece	69	24	235	3	8	3.1	2.8	1.1	40	41	72	1.0	90	100	.07	.10	.6	Trace
393	Cupcake, 2 1/2-in diam. 1 cupcake	35	24	120	2	4	1.6	1.4	.5	20	21	37	.5	46	50	.03	.05	.3	Trace

Column headers as printed: (A) item number · (B) food and approximate measure · measure · (C)–(T) nutrient values.

No.	Food and approximate measure	Measure	(C)	(D)	(E)	(F)	(G)	(H)	(I)	(J)	(K)	(L)	(M)	(N)	(O)	(P)	(Q)	(R)	(S)	(T)
	Gingerbread:																			
394	Whole cake (8-in square)	1 cake	570	37	1,575	18	39	9.7	16.6	10.0	291	513	570	8.6	1,562	Trace	0.84	1.00	7.4	Trace
395	Piece, 1/9 of cake	1 piece	63	37	175	2	4	1.1	1.8	1.1	32	57	63	.9	173	Trace	.09	.11	.8	Trace
	White, 2 layer with chocolate icing:																			
396	Whole cake (8- or 9-in diam.)	1 cake	1,140	21	4,000	44	122	48.2	46.4	20.0	716	1,129	2,041	11.4	1,322	680	1.50	1.77	12.5	2
397	Piece, 1/16 of cake	1 piece	71	21	250	3	8	3.0	2.9	1.2	45	70	127	.7	82	40	.09	.11	.8	Trace
	Yellow, 2 layer with chocolate icing:																			
398	Whole cake (8- or 9-in diam.)	1 cake	1,108	26	3,735	45	125	47.8	47.8	20.3	638	1,008	2,017	12.2	1,208	1,550	1.24	1.67	10.6	2
399	Piece, 1/16 of cake	1 piece	69	26	235	3	8	3.0	3.0	1.3	40	63	126	.8	75	100	.08	.10	.7	Trace
	Cakes made from home recipes using enriched flour:[*] **Boston cream pie with custard filling:**																			
400	Whole cake (8-in diam.)	1 cake	825	35	2,490	41	78	23.0	30.1	15.2	412	553	833	8.2	*734	1,730	1.04	1.27	9.6	2
401	Piece, 1/12 of cake	1 piece	69	35	210	3	6	1.9	2.5	1.3	34	46	70	.7	*61	140	.09	.11	.8	Trace
	Fruitcake, dark:																			
402	Loaf, 1-lb (7 1/2 by 2 by 1 1/2 in)	1 loaf	454	18	1,720	22	69	14.4	33.5	14.8	271	327	513	11.8	2,250	540	.72	.73	4.9	2
403	Slice, 1/30 of loaf	1 slice	15	18	55	1	2	.5	1.1	.5	9	11	17	.4	74	20	.02	.02	.2	Trace
	Plain, sheet cake: Without icing:																			
404	Whole cake (9-in square)	1 cake	777	25	2,830	35	108	29.5	44.4	23.9	434	497	793	8.5	*614	1,320	1.21	1.40	10.2	2
405	Piece, 1/9 of cake	1 piece	86	25	315	4	12	3.3	4.9	2.6	48	55	88	.9	*68	150	.13	.15	1.1	Trace
	With uncooked white icing:																			
406	Whole cake (9-in square)	1 cake	1,096	21	4,020	37	129	42.2	49.5	24.4	694	548	822	8.2	*669	2,190	1.22	1.47	10.2	2
407	Piece, 1/9 of cake	1 piece	121	21	445	4	14	4.7	5.5	2.7	77	61	91	.8	*74	240	.14	.16	1.1	Trace
	Pound:[**]																			
408	Loaf, 8 1/2 by 3 1/2 by 3 1/4 in.	1 loaf	565	16	2,725	31	170	42.9	73.1	39.6	273	107	418	7.9	345	1,410	.90	.99	7.3	0
409	Slice, 1/17 of loaf	1 slice	33	16	160	2	10	2.5	4.3	2.3	16	6	24	.5	20	80	.05	.06	.4	0
	Sponge cake:																			
410	Whole cake (9 3/4-in diam. tube cake)	1 cake	790	32	2,345	60	45	13.1	15.8	5.7	427	237	885	13.4	687	3,560	1.10	1.64	7.4	Trace
411	Piece, 1/12 of cake	1 piece	66	32	195	5	4	1.1	1.3	.5	36	20	74	1.1	57	300	.09	.14	.6	Trace
	Cookies made with enriched flour:[33] **Brownies with nuts: Home-prepared, 1 3/4 by 1 3/4 by 7/8 in:**																			
412	From home recipe	1 brownie	20	10	95	1	6	1.5	3.0	1.2	10	8	30	.4	38	40	.04	.03	.2	Trace
413	From commercial recipe	1 brownie	20	11	85	1	4	.9	1.4	1.3	13	9	27	.4	34	20	.03	.02	.2	Trace
414	Frozen, with chocolate icing,[11] 1 1/2 by 1 3/4 by 7/8 in.	1 brownie	25	13	105	1	5	2.0	2.2	.7	15	10	31	.4	44	50	.03	.03	.2	Trace
	Chocolate chip:																			
415	Commercial, 2 1/4-in diam., 3/8 in thick	4 cookies	42	3	200	2	9	2.8	2.9	2.2	29	16	48	1.0	56	50	.10	.17	.9	Trace
416	From home recipe, 2 1/3-in diam.	4 cookies	40	3	205	2	12	3.5	4.5	2.9	24	14	40	.8	47	40	.06	.06	.5	Trace
417	Fig bars, square (1 5/8 by 1 5/8 by 3/8 in) or rectangular (1 1/2 by 1 3/4 by 1/2 in)	4 cookies	56	14	200	2	3	.8	1.2	.7	42	44	34	1.0	111	60	.04	.14	.9	Trace
418	Gingersnaps, 2-in diam., 1/4 in thick	4 cookies	28	3	90	2	2	.7	.7	.6	22	20	13	.7	129	20	.08	.06	.7	0
419	Macaroons, 2 3/4-in diam., 1/4 in thick	2 cookies	38	4	180	2	9	—	—	—	25	10	32	.3	176	0	.02	.06	.2	0
420	Oatmeal with raisins, 2 5/8-in diam., 1/4 in thick	4 cookies	52	3	235	3	8	2.0	3.3	2.0	38	11	53	1.4	192	30	.15	.10	1.0	Trace

*Value varies with the brand. Consult the label.
**Value varies with the brand. Consult the label.
Applies to product with added ascorbic acid. Without added ascorbic acid, value is trace.
Applies to product with added ascorbic acid.
Excepting angelfood cake. Without added ascorbic acid, value would be higher.
Excepting spongecake, vegetable shortening used for cake portion; butter, for icing. If butter or margarine used for cake portion, vitamin A values would be higher.
Applies to product made with a sodium aluminum-sulfate type baking powder. With a low-sodium type baking powder containing potassium, value would be about twice the amount shown.
Equal weights of flour, sugar, eggs, and vegetable shortening.
Products are commercial.
Made with enriched flour and vegetable shortening except for macaroons which do not contain flour or shortening.
Icing made with butter.

(A)	(B)	(C) Grams	Per cent	(D) Calories	(E) Grams	(F) Grams	(G) Grams	(H) Grams	(I) Grams	(J) Grams	(K) Milligrams	(L) Milligrams	(M) Milligrams	(N) Milligrams	(O) International units	(P) Milligrams	(Q) Milligrams	(R) Milligrams	(S) Milligrams
	GRAIN PRODUCTS—Con.																		
	Cookies made with enriched flour⁵¹—Continued																		
421	Plain, prepared from commercial chilled dough, 2 1/2-in diam. 1/4 in thick. 4 cookies	48	5	240	2	12	3.0	5.2	2.9	31	17	35	0.6	23	30	0.10	0.08	0.9	0
422	Sandwich type (chocolate or vanilla), 1 3/4-in diam. 3/8-in thick. 4 cookies	40	2	200	2	9	2.2	3.9	2.2	28	10	96	.7	15	0	.06	.10	.7	0
423	Vanilla wafers, 1 3/4-in diam. 1/4 in thick. 10 cookies	40	3	185	2	6	.5	—	—	30	16	25	.6	29	50	.10	.09	.8	0
	Cornmeal:																		
424	Whole-ground, unbolted, dry form. 1 cup	122	12	435	11	5	.5	1.0	2.5	90	24	312	2.9	346	⁵620	.46	.13	2.4	0
425	Bolted (nearly whole-grain), dry form. 1 cup	122	12	440	11	4	.5	.9	2.1	91	21	272	2.2	303	⁵590	.37	.10	2.3	0
	Degermed, enriched:																		
426	Dry form. 1 cup	138	12	500	11	2	.2	.4	.9	108	8	137	4.0	166	⁵1140	.61	.36	4.8	0
427	Cooked. 1 cup	240	88	120	3	Trace	Trace	.1	.2	26	2	34	1.0	38	⁵140	.14	.10	1.2	0
	Degermed, unenriched:																		
428	Dry form. 1 cup	138	12	500	11	2	.2	.4	.9	108	8	137	1.5	166	⁵1610	.19	.07	1.4	0
429	Cooked. 1 cup	240	88	120	3	Trace	Trace	.1	.2	26	2	34	.5	38	⁵140	.05	.02	.2	0
	Crackers:³⁸																		
430	Graham, plain, 2 1/2-in square. 2 crackers	14	6	55	1	1	.3	.5	.3	10	6	21	.5	55	0	.02	.08	.5	0
431	Rye wafers, whole-grain, 1 7/8 by 3 1/2 in. 2 wafers	13	6	45	2	Trace	—	—	—	10	7	50	.5	78	0	.04	.03	.2	0
432	Saltines, made with enriched flour. 4 crackers or 1 packet	11	4	50	1	1	.3	.5	.4	8	2	10	.5	13	0	.05	.05	.4	0
	Danish pastry (enriched flour), plain without fruit or nuts:³⁸																		
433	Packaged ring, 12 oz. 1 ring	340	22	1,435	25	80	24.3	31.7	16.5	155	170	371	6.1	381	1,050	.97	1.01	8.6	Trace
434	Round piece, about 4 1/4-in. 1 pastry	65	22	275	5	15	4.7	6.1	3.2	30	33	71	1.2	73	200	.18	.19	1.7	Trace
435	Ounce. 1 oz	28	22	120	2	7	2.0	2.7	1.4	13	14	31	.5	32	90	.08	.08	.7	Trace
	Doughnuts, made with enriched flour:³⁸																		
436	Cake type, plain, 2 1/2-in diam. 1 in high. 1 doughnut	25	24	100	1	5	1.2	2.0	1.1	13	10	48	.4	23	20	.05	.05	.4	Trace
437	Yeast-leavened, glazed, 3 3/4-in diam. 1 1/4 in high. 1 doughnut	50	26	205	3	11	3.3	5.8	3.3	22	16	33	.6	34	25	.10	.10	.8	0
	Macaroni, enriched, cooked (cut lengths, elbows, shells):																		
438	Firm stage (hot). 1 cup	130	64	190	7	1	—	—	—	39	14	85	1.4	103	0	.23	.13	1.8	0
	Tender stage:																		
439	Cold macaroni. 1 cup	105	73	115	4	Trace	—	—	—	24	8	53	.9	64	0	.15	.08	1.2	0
440	Hot macaroni. 1 cup	140	73	155	5	1	—	—	—	32	11	70	1.3	85	0	.20	.11	1.5	0
	Macaroni (enriched) and cheese:																		
441	Canned.³⁹ 1 cup	240	80	230	9	10	4.2	3.1	1.4	26	199	182	1.0	139	260	.12	.24	1.0	Trace
442	From home recipe (served hot).³⁸ 1 cup	200	58	430	17	22	8.9	8.8	2.9	40	362	322	1.8	240	860	.20	.40	1.8	Trace
	Muffins made with enriched flour:³⁸																		
443	Blueberry, 2 3/8-in diam. 1 1/2 in high. 1 muffin	40	39	110	3	4	1.1	1.4	.7	17	34	53	.6	46	90	.09	.10	.7	Trace
444	Bran. 1 muffin	40	35	105	3	4	1.2	1.4	.8	17	57	162	1.5	172	90	.07	.10	1.7	Trace
445	Corn (enriched degermed cornmeal and flour), 2 3/8-in diam. 1 1/2 in high. 1 muffin	40	33	125	3	4	1.2	1.6	.9	19	42	168	.7	54	⁵120	.10	.10	.7	Trace

(A)	(B)	Measure	g	(C)	(D)	(E)	(F)	(G)	(H)	(I)	(J)	(K)	(L)	(M)	(N)	(O)	(P)	(Q)	(R)	(S)
446	Plain, 3-in diam., 1 1/2 in high.	1 muffin	40	38	120	3	4	1.0	1.7	1.0	17	42	60	0.6	50	40	.09	.12	0.9	Trace
447	From mix, egg, milk: Corn, 2 3/8-in diam., 1 1/2 in high.[54]	1 muffin	40	30	130	3	4	1.2	1.7	.9	20	96	152	.6	44	[57]100	.08	.09	.7	Trace
448	Noodles (egg noodles), enriched, cooked.	1 cup	160	71	200	7	2	—	—	—	37	16	94	1.4	70	110	.22	.13	1.9	0
449	Noodles, chow mein, canned.	1 cup	45	1	220	6	11	—	—	—	26	—	—	—	—	—	—	—	—	0
450	Pancakes, (4-in diam.):[55] Buckwheat, made from mix (with buckwheat and enriched flours), egg and milk added.	1 cake	27	58	55	2	2	.8	.9	.4	6	59	91	.4	66	60	.04	.05	.2	Trace
451	Plain: Made from home recipe using enriched flour.	1 cake	27	50	60	2	2	.5	.8	.5	9	27	38	.4	33	30	.06	.07	.5	Trace
452	Made from mix with enriched flour, egg and milk added.	1 cake	27	51	60	2	2	.7	.7	.3	9	58	70	.3	42	70	.04	.06	.2	Trace
	Pies, piecrust made with enriched flour, vegetable shortening (9-in diam.): Apple:																			
453	Whole	1 pie	945	48	2,420	21	105	27.0	44.5	25.2	360	76	208	6.6	756	280	1.06	.79	9.3	9
454	Sector, 1/7 of pie	1 sector	135	48	345	3	15	3.9	6.4	3.6	51	11	30	.9	108	40	.15	.11	1.3	2
	Banana cream:																			
455	Whole	1 pie	910	54	2,010	41	85	26.7	33.2	16.2	279	601	746	7.3	1,847	2,280	.77	1.51	7.0	9
456	Sector, 1/7 of pie	1 sector	130	54	285	6	12	3.8	4.7	2.3	40	86	107	1.0	264	330	.11	.22	1.0	1
	Blueberry:																			
457	Whole	1 pie	945	51	2,285	23	102	24.8	43.7	25.1	330	104	217	9.5	614	280	1.03	.80	10.0	28
458	Sector, 1/7 of pie	1 sector	135	51	325	3	15	3.5	6.2	3.6	47	15	31	1.4	88	40	.15	.11	1.4	4
	Cherry:																			
459	Whole	1 pie	945	47	2,465	25	107	28.2	45.0	25.3	363	132	236	6.6	992	4,160	1.09	.84	9.8	Trace
460	Sector, 1/7 of pie	1 sector	135	47	350	4	15	4.0	6.4	3.6	52	19	34	.9	142	590	.16	.12	1.4	Trace
	Custard:																			
461	Whole	1 pie	910	58	1,985	56	101	33.9	38.5	17.5	213	874	1,028	8.2	1,247	2,090	.79	1.92	5.6	0
462	Sector, 1/7 of pie	1 sector	130	58	285	8	14	4.8	5.5	2.5	30	125	147	1.2	178	300	.11	.27	.8	0
	Lemon meringue:																			
463	Whole	1 pie	840	47	2,140	31	86	26.1	33.8	16.4	317	118	412	6.7	420	1,430	.61	.84	5.2	25
464	Sector, 1/7 of pie	1 sector	120	47	305	4	12	3.7	4.8	2.3	45	17	59	1.0	60	200	.09	.12	.7	4
	Mince:																			
465	Whole	1 pie	945	43	2,560	24	109	28.0	45.9	25.2	389	265	359	13.3	1,682	20	.96	.86	9.8	9
466	Sector, 1/7 of pie	1 sector	135	43	365	3	16	4.0	6.6	3.6	56	38	51	1.9	240	Trace	.14	.12	1.4	1
	Peach:																			
467	Whole	1 pie	945	48	2,410	24	101	24.8	43.7	25.1	361	95	274	8.5	1,408	6,900	1.04	.97	14.0	28
468	Sector, 1/7 of pie	1 sector	135	48	345	3	14	3.5	6.2	3.6	52	14	39	1.2	201	990	.15	.14	2.0	4
	Pecan:																			
469	Whole	1 pie	825	20	3,450	42	189	27.8	101.0	44.2	423	388	850	25.6	1,015	1,320	1.80	.95	6.9	Trace
470	Sector, 1/7 of pie	1 sector	118	20	495	6	27	4.0	14.4	6.3	61	55	122	3.7	145	190	.26	.14	1.0	Trace
	Pumpkin:																			
471	Whole	1 pie	910	59	1,920	36	102	37.4	37.5	16.6	223	464	628	7.3	1,456	22,480	.78	1.27	7.0	Trace
472	Sector, 1/7 of pie	1 sector	130	59	275	5	15	5.4	5.4	2.4	32	66	90	1.0	208	3,210	.11	.18	1.0	Trace
473	Piecrust (home recipe) made with enriched flour and vegetable shortening, baked.	1 pie shell, 9-in diam.	180	15	900	11	60	14.8	26.1	14.9	79	25	90	3.1	89	0	.47	.40	5.0	0
474	Piecrust mix with enriched flour and vegetable shortening, 10-oz pkg. prepared and baked.	Piecrust for 2-crust pie, 9-in diam.	320	19	1,485	20	93	22.7	39.7	23.4	141	131	272	6.1	179	0	1.07	.79	9.9	0

[54] Made with vegetable shortening.
[55] Products are commercial unless otherwise specified.
[56] Made with enriched flour and vegetable shortening except for macaroons which do not contain flour or shortening.
[57] Applies to yellow varieties; white varieties contain only a trace.
[58] Contains vegetable shortening and butter.
[59] Made with corn oil.
[60] Made with regular margarine.
[61] Applies to product made with yellow cornmeal.
[62] Made with enriched degermed cornmeal and enriched flour.

(A)	(B)	Grams	(C) Per-cent	(D) Cal-ories	(E) Grams	(F) Grams	(G) Grams	(H) Grams	(I) Grams	(J) Grams	(K) Milli-grams	(L) Milli-grams	(M) Milli-grams	(N) Milli-grams	(O) Inter-national units	(P) Milli-grams	(Q) Milli-grams	(R) Milli-grams	(S) Milli-grams
	GRAIN PRODUCTS—Con.																		
475	Pizza (cheese) baked, 4 3/4-in sector; 1/8 of 12-in pie.[13]	1 sector	60	45	145	6	4	1.7	1.5	0.6	22	86	89	1.1	67	230	0.16	0.18	1.6	4
	Popcorn, popped:																		
476	Plain, large kernel	1 cup	6	4	25	1	Trace	Trace	.1	.2	5	1	17	.2	—	—	—	.01	.1	0
477	With oil (coconut) and salt added, large kernel.	1 cup	9	3	40	1	2	1.5	.2	.2	5	1	19	.2	—	—	—	.01	.2	0
478	Sugar coated	1 cup	35	4	135	2	1	.5	.2	.4	30	2	47	.5	—	—	.02	.4	0	
	Pretzels, made with enriched flour:																		
479	Dutch, twisted, 2 3/4 by 2 5/8 in.	1 pretzel	16	5	60	2	1	—	—	—	12	4	21	.2	21	0	.05	.04	.7	0
480	Thin, twisted, 3 1/4 by 2 1/4 by 1/4 in.	10 pretzels	60	5	235	6	3	—	—	—	46	13	79	.9	78	0	.20	.15	2.5	0
481	Stick, 2 1/4 in long	10 pretzels	3	5	10	Trace	Trace	—	—	—	2	1	4	Trace	4	0	.01	.01	.1	0
	Rice, white, enriched:																		
	Long grain:																		
482	Raw	1 cup	165	73	180	4	Trace	Trace	Trace	Trace	40	5	31	1.3	31	0	.21	(55)	1.7	0
483	Cooked, served hot	1 cup	185	12	670	14	1	.2	.1	.2	149	44	174	5.4	170	0	.81	.06	6.5	0
484	Parboiled: Raw	1 cup	205	73	225	4	Trace	.1	.1	.1	50	21	57	1.8	57	0	.23	.02	2.1	0
485	Raw	1 cup	185	10	685	14	1	.2	.1	.2	150	111	370	5.4	278	0	.81	.07	6.5	0
486	Cooked, served hot[38]	1 cup	175	73	185	4	Trace	.1	.1	.1	41	33	100	1.4	75	0	.19	.02	2.1	0
	Rolls, enriched:[38]																		
	Commercial:																		
487	Brown-and-serve (12 per 12-oz pkg.), browned.	1 roll	26	27	85	2	2	.4	.7	.5	14	20	23	.5	25	Trace	.10	.06	.9	Trace
488	Cloverleaf or pan, 2 1/2-in diam., 2 in high.	1 roll	28	31	85	2	2	.4	.6	.4	15	21	21	.5	27	Trace	.11	.07	.9	Trace
489	Frankfurter and hamburger (8 per 11 1/2-oz pkg.).	1 roll	40	31	120	3	2	.5	.8	.6	21	30	34	.8	38	Trace	.16	.10	1.3	Trace
490	Hard, 3 3/4-in diam., 2 in high.	1 roll	50	25	155	5	2	.4	.6	.5	30	24	46	1.2	49	Trace	.20	.12	1.7	Trace
491	Hoagie or submarine, 11 1/2 by 3 by 2 1/2 in.	1 roll	135	31	390	12	4	.9	1.4	1.4	75	58	115	3.0	122	Trace	.54	.32	4.5	Trace
	From home recipe:																		
492	Cloverleaf, 2 1/2-in diam., 2 in high.	1 roll	35	26	120	3	3	.8	1.1	.7	20	16	36	.7	41	30	.12	.12	1.2	Trace
	Spaghetti, enriched, cooked:																		
493	Firm stage, "al dente," served hot.	1 cup	130	64	190	7	1	—	—	—	39	14	85	1.4	103	0	.23	.13	1.8	0
494	Tender stage, served hot	1 cup	140	73	155	5	1	—	—	—	32	11	70	1.3	85	0	.20	.11	1.5	0
	Spaghetti (enriched) in tomato sauce with cheese:																		
495	From home recipe	1 cup	250	77	260	9	9	2.0	5.4	.7	37	80	135	2.3	408	1,080	.25	.18	2.3	13
496	Canned	1 cup	250	80	190	6	2	.5	.3	.4	39	40	88	2.8	303	930	.35	.28	4.5	10
	Spaghetti (enriched) with meat balls and tomato sauce:																		
497	From home recipe	1 cup	248	70	330	19	12	3.3	6.3	.9	39	124	236	3.7	665	1,590	.25	.30	4.0	22
498	Canned	1 cup	250	78	260	12	10	2.2	3.3	3.9	29	53	113	3.3	245	1,000	.15	.18	2.3	5
499	Toaster pastries	1 pastry	50	12	200	3	6	—	—	—	36	[54]	[67]	1.9	[74]	500	.16	.17	2.1	(40)
	Waffles, made with enriched flour, 7-in diam.:[18]																		
500	From home recipe	1 waffle	75	41	210	7	7	2.3	2.8	1.4	28	85	130	1.3	109	250	.17	.23	1.4	Trace
501	From mix, egg and milk added	1 waffle	75	42	205	7	8	2.8	2.9	1.2	27	179	257	1.0	146	170	.14	.22	.9	Trace

The following table gives nutritive values. Columns are lettered (A) through (S): (A) item number; (B) food, approximate measure; (C) grams; (D) water (%); (E) food energy (calories); (F) protein (g); (G) fat (g); (H) saturated fatty acids (g); (I) oleic (g); (J) linoleic (g); (K) carbohydrate (g); (L) calcium (mg); (M) iron (mg); (N) potassium (mg); (O) vitamin A (IU); (P) thiamin (mg); (Q) riboflavin (mg); (R) niacin (mg); (S) ascorbic acid (mg).

(A)	(B)	(C)	(D)	(E)	(F)	(G)	(H)	(I)	(J)	(K)	(L)	(M)	(N)	(O)	(P)	(Q)	(R)	(S)
	Wheat flours:																	
	All-purpose or family flour.																	
	Enriched:																	
502	Sifted, spooned----------- 1 cup	115	12	420	12	1	0.2	0.1	0.5	88	18	3.3	109	0	0.74	0.46	6.1	0
503	Unsifted, spooned--------- 1 cup	125	12	455	13	1	.2	.1	.5	95	20	3.6	119	0	.80	.50	6.6	0
504	Cake or pastry flour, enriched, sifted, spooned. 1 cup	96	12	350	7	1	.1	.1	.3	76	16	2.8	91	0	.61	.38	5.1	0
505	Self-rising, enriched, unsifted, spooned. 1 cup	125	12	440	12	1	.2	.1	.5	93	331	3.6	—	0	.80	.50	6.6	0
506	Whole-wheat, from hard wheats, stirred. 1 cup	120	12	400	16	2	.4	.2	1.0	85	49	4.0	444	0	.66	.14	5.2	0
	LEGUMES (DRY), NUTS, SEEDS; RELATED PRODUCTS																	
	Almonds, shelled:																	
507	Chopped (about 130 almonds)- 1 cup	130	5	775	24	70	5.6	47.7	12.8	25	304	6.1	1,005	0	.31	1.20	4.6	Trace
508	Slivered, not pressed down (about 115 almonds). 1 cup	115	5	690	21	62	5.0	42.2	11.3	22	269	5.4	889	0	.28	1.06	4.0	Trace
	Beans, dry:																	
	Common varieties as Great Northern, navy, and others:																	
	Cooked, drained:																	
509	Great Northern------------ 1 cup	180	69	210	14	1	—	—	—	38	90	4.9	749	0	.25	.13	1.3	0
510	Pea (navy)---------------- 1 cup	190	69	225	15	1	—	—	—	40	95	5.1	790	0	.27	.13	1.3	0
	Canned, solids and liquid:																	
	White with—																	
511	Frankfurters (sliced)----- 1 cup	255	71	365	19	18				32	94	4.8	668	330	.18	.15	3.3	Trace
512	Pork and tomato sauce----- 1 cup	255	71	310	16	7	2.4	2.8	.6	48	138	4.6	536	330	.20	.08	1.5	5
513	Pork and sweet sauce------ 1 cup	255	66	385	16	12	4.3	5.0	1.1	54	161	5.9	—	—	.15	.10	1.3	—
514	Red kidney---------------- 1 cup	255	76	230	15	1	—	—	—	42	74	4.6	673	10	.13	.10	1.5	—
515	Lima, cooked, drained----- 1 cup	190	64	260	16	1	—	—	—	49	55	5.9	1,163	—	.25	.11	1.3	—
516	Blackeye peas, dry cooked (with residual cooking liquid). 1 cup	250	80	190	13	1	—	—	—	35	43	3.3	573	30	.40	.10	1.0	—
517	Brazil nuts, shelled (6-8 large kernels). 1 oz	28	5	185	4	19	4.8	6.2	7.1	3	53	1.0	203	Trace	.27	.03	.5	—
518	Cashew nuts, roasted in oil- 1 cup	140	5	785	24	64	12.9	36.8	10.2	41	53	5.3	650	140	.60	.35	2.5	—
	Coconut meat, fresh:																	
519	Piece, about 2 by 2 by 1/2 in- 1 piece	45	51	155	2	16	14.0	.9	.3	4	6	.8	115	0	.02	.01	.2	1
520	Shredded or grated, not pressed down. 1 cup	80	51	275	3	28	24.8	1.6	.5	8	10	1.4	205	0	.04	.02	.4	2
521	Filberts (hazelnuts), chopped (about 80 kernels). 1 cup	115	6	730	14	72	5.1	55.2	7.3	19	240	3.9	810	—	.53	—	1.0	Trace
522	Lentils, whole, cooked----- 1 cup	200	72	210	16	Trace	—	—	—	39	50	4.2	498	40	.14	.12	1.2	0
523	Peanuts, roasted in oil, salted (whole, halves, chopped). 1 cup	144	2	840	37	72	13.7	33.0	20.7	27	107	3.0	971	—	.46	.19	24.8	0
524	Peanut butter------------- 1 tbsp	16	2	95	4	8	1.5	3.7	2.3	3	9	.3	100	—	.02	.02	2.4	0
525	Peas, split, dry, cooked--- 1 cup	200	70	230	16	1	—	—	—	42	22	3.4	592	80	.30	.18	1.8	—
526	Pecans, chopped or pieces (about 120 large halves). 1 cup	118	3	810	11	84	7.2	50.5	20.0	17	86	2.8	712	150	1.01	.15	1.1	2
527	Pumpkin and squash kernels, dry, hulled. 1 cup	140	4	775	41	65	11.8	23.5	27.5	21	71	15.7	1,386	100	.34	.27	3.4	—
528	Sunflower seeds, dry, hulled- 1 cup	145	5	810	35	69	8.2	13.7	43.2	29	174	10.3	1,334	70	2.84	.33	7.8	—
	Walnuts:																	
	Black:																	
529	Chopped or broken kernels-- 1 cup	125	3	785	26	74	6.3	13.3	45.7	19	Trace	7.5	575	380	.28	.14	.9	—
530	Ground (finely)----------- 1 cup	80	3	500	16	47	4.0	8.5	29.2	12	Trace	4.8	368	240	.18	.09	.6	—
531	Persian or English, chopped (about 60 halves). 1 cup	120	4	780	18	77	8.4	11.8	42.2	19	119	3.7	540	40	.40	.16	1.1	2

[57] Crust made with vegetable shortening and enriched flour.
[58] Made with vegetable shortening.
[59] Product may or may not be enriched with riboflavin. Consult the label.
[60] Value varies with the brand. Consult the label.

SUGARS AND SWEETS

(A)	(B)	Grams	(C) Per cent	(D) Cal-ories	(E) Grams	(F) Grams	(G) Grams	(H) Grams	(I) Grams	(J) Grams	(K) Milli-grams	(L) Milli-grams	(M) Milli-grams	(N) Milli-grams	(O) Inter-national units	(P) Milli-grams	(Q) Milli-grams	(R) Milli-grams	(S) Milli-grams
	Cake icings:																		
	Boiled, white:																		
532	Plain — 1 cup	94	18	295	1	0	0	0	0	75	2	2	Trace	17	0	Trace	0.03	Trace	0
533	With coconut — 1 cup	166	15	605	3	13	11.0	.9	Trace	124	10	50	0.8	277	0	0.02	.07	0.3	0
	Uncooked:																		
534	Chocolate made with milk and butter — 1 cup	275	14	1,035	9	38	23.4	11.7	1.0	185	165	305	3.3	536	580	.06	.28	.6	1
535	Creamy fudge from mix and water — 1 cup	245	15	830	7	16	5.1	6.7	3.1	183	96	218	2.7	238	Trace	.05	.20	.7	Trace
536	White — 1 cup	319	11	1,200	2	21	12.7	5.1	.5	260	48	38	Trace	57	860	Trace	.06	Trace	Trace
	Candy:																		
537	Caramels, plain or chocolate — 1 oz	28	8	115	1	3	1.6	1.1	.1	22	42	35	.4	54	Trace	.01	.05	.1	Trace
	Chocolate:																		
538	Milk, plain — 1 oz	28	1	145	2	9	5.5	3.0	.3	16	65	65	.3	109	80	.02	.10	.1	Trace
539	Semisweet, small pieces (60 per oz) — 1 cup or 6-oz pkg	170	1	860	7	61	36.2	19.8	1.7	97	51	255	4.4	553	30	.02	.14	.9	0
540	Chocolate-coated peanuts — 1 oz	28	1	160	5	12	4.0	4.7	2.1	11	33	84	.4	143	Trace	.10	.05	2.1	Trace
541	Fondant, uncoated (mints, candy corn, other) — 1 oz	28	8	105	Trace	Trace	.1	.3	.1	25	4	2	.3	1	0	Trace	Trace	Trace	0
542	Fudge, chocolate, plain — 1 oz	28	8	115	1	3	1.3	1.4	.6	21	22	24	.3	42	Trace	.01	.03	.1	Trace
543	Gum drops — 1 oz	28	12	100	Trace	Trace	—	—	—	25	2	Trace	.1	1	0	0	Trace	Trace	0
544	Hard — 1 oz	28	1	110	0	Trace	—	—	—	28	6	2	.5	1	0	0	0	0	0
545	Marshmallows — 1 oz	28	17	90	1	Trace	—	—	—	23	5	2	.5	2	0	0	Trace	Trace	0
	Chocolate-flavored beverage powders (about 4 heaping tsp per oz):																		
546	With nonfat dry milk — 1 oz	28	2	100	5	1	.5	.3	Trace	20	167	155	.5	227	10	.04	.21	.2	1
547	Without milk — 1 oz	28	1	100	1	1	.4	.2	Trace	25	9	48	.6	142	0	.01	.03	.1	Trace
548	Honey, strained or extracted — 1 tbsp	21	17	65	Trace	0	0	0	—	17	1	4	.1	11	0	Trace	.01	.1	Trace
549	Jams and preserves — 1 tbsp	20	29	55	Trace	Trace	—	—	—	14	4	2	.2	18	Trace	Trace	.01	Trace	Trace
550	1 packet	14	29	40	Trace	Trace	—	—	—	10	3	1	.3	12	Trace	Trace	.01	Trace	1
551	Jellies — 1 tbsp	18	29	50	Trace	Trace	—	—	—	13	4	1	.2	14	Trace	Trace	.01	Trace	Trace
552	1 packet	14	29	40	Trace	Trace	—	—	—	10	3	1	.2	11	Trace	Trace	Trace	Trace	1
	Sirups:																		
	Chocolate-flavored sirup or topping:																		
553	Thin type — 1 fl oz or 2 tbsp	38	32	90	1	1	.5	.3	Trace	24	6	35	.6	106	Trace	.01	.03	.2	0
554	Fudge type — 1 fl oz or 2 tbsp	38	25	125	2	5	3.1	1.6	.1	20	48	60	.5	107	60	.02	.08	.2	Trace
	Molasses, cane:																		
555	Light (first extraction) — 1 tbsp	20	24	50	—	—	—	—	—	13	33	—	.9	183	—	.01	.01	Trace	—
556	Blackstrap (third extraction) — 1 tbsp	20	24	45	—	—	—	—	—	11	137	—	3.2	585	—	.02	.04	.4	—
557	Sorghum — 1 tbsp	21	23	55	—	—	—	—	—	14	35	—	2.6	—	—	—	.02	Trace	—
558	Table blends, chiefly corn, light and dark — 1 tbsp	21	24	60	0	0	0	0	0	15	9	3	.8	1	0	0	0	0	0
559	Sugars: Brown, pressed down — 1 cup	220	2	820	0	0	0	0	0	212	187	42	7.5	757	0	.02	.07	.4	0
	White:																		
560	Granulated — 1 cup	200	1	770	0	0	0	0	0	199	0	0	.2	6	0	0	0	0	0
561	1 tbsp	12	1	45	0	0	0	0	0	12	0	0	Trace	Trace	0	0	0	0	0
562	1 packet	6	1	23	0	0	0	0	0	6	0	0	Trace	Trace	0	0	0	0	0
563	Powdered, sifted, spooned into cup — 1 cup	100	1	385	0	0	0	0	0	100	0	0	.1	3	0	0	0	0	0

VEGETABLE AND VEGETABLE PRODUCTS

(A)	(B)	(C)	(D)	(E)	(F)	(G)	(H)	(I)	(J)	(K)	(L)	(M)	(N)	(O)	(P)	(Q)	(R)	(S)
	Asparagus, green:																	
	Cooked, drained:																	
	Cuts and tips, 1 1/2- to 2-in lengths:																	
564	From raw— 1 cup — 145	94	30	3	Trace	---	---	---	5	30	73	0.9	265	1,310	0.23	0.26	2.0	38
565	From frozen— 1 cup — 180	93	40	6	Trace	---	---	---	6	40	115	2.2	396	1,530	.25	.23	1.8	41
	Spears, 1/2-in diam. at base:																	
566	From raw— 4 spears — 60	94	10	1	Trace	---	---	---	2	13	30	.4	110	540	.10	.11	.8	16
567	From frozen— 4 spears — 60	92	15	2	Trace	---	---	---	2	13	40	.7	143	470	.10	.08	.7	16
568	Canned, spears, 1/2-in diam. at base. 4 spears — 80	93	15	2	Trace	---	---	---	3	15	42	1.5	133	640	.05	.08	.6	12
	Beans:																	
	Lima, immature seeds, frozen, cooked, drained:																	
569	Thick-seeded types (Fordhooks) 1 cup — 170	74	170	10	Trace	---	---	---	32	34	153	2.9	724	390	.12	.09	1.7	29
570	Thin-seeded types (baby limas) 1 cup — 180	69	210	13	Trace	---	---	---	40	63	227	4.7	709	400	.16	.09	2.2	22
	Snap:																	
	Green:																	
	Cooked, drained:																	
571	From raw (cuts and French style) 1 cup — 125	92	30	2	Trace	---	---	---	7	63	46	.8	189	680	.09	.11	.6	15
	From frozen:																	
572	Cuts— 1 cup — 135	92	35	2	Trace	---	---	---	8	54	43	.9	205	780	.09	.12	.5	7
573	French style— 1 cup — 130	92	35	2	Trace	---	---	---	8	49	39	1.2	177	690	.08	.10	.4	9
574	Canned, drained solids (cuts) 1 cup — 135	92	30	2	Trace	---	---	---	7	61	34	2.0	128	630	.04	.07	.4	5
	Yellow or wax:																	
	Cooked, drained:																	
575	From raw (cuts and French style) 1 cup — 125	93	30	2	Trace	---	---	---	6	63	46	.8	189	290	.09	.11	.6	16
	From frozen (cuts):																	
576	From frozen (cuts) 1 cup — 135	92	35	2	Trace	---	---	---	8	47	42	.9	221	140	.09	.11	.5	8
577	Canned, drained solids (cuts) 1 cup — 135	92	30	2	Trace	---	---	---	7	61	34	2.0	128	140	.04	.07	.4	7
	Beans, mature. See Beans, dry (items 509-515) and Blackeye peas (item 516).																	
	Bean sprouts (mung):																	
578	Raw— 1 cup — 105	89	35	4	Trace	---	---	---	7	20	67	1.4	234	20	.14	.14	.8	20
579	Cooked, drained— 1 cup — 125	91	35	4	Trace	---	---	---	7	21	60	1.1	195	30	.11	.13	.9	8
	Beets:																	
	Cooked, drained, peeled:																	
580	Whole beets, 2-in diam.— 2 beets — 100	91	30	1	Trace	---	---	---	7	14	23	.5	208	20	.03	.04	.3	6
581	Diced or sliced— 1 cup — 170	91	55	2	Trace	---	---	---	12	24	39	.9	354	30	.05	.07	.5	10
	Canned, drained solids:																	
582	Whole beets, small— 1 cup — 160	89	60	2	Trace	---	---	---	14	32	29	1.1	267	30	.02	.05	.2	5
583	Diced or sliced— 1 cup — 170	89	65	2	Trace	---	---	---	15	32	31	1.2	284	30	.02	.05	.2	5
584	Beet greens, leaves and stems, cooked, drained. 1 cup — 145	94	25	2	Trace	---	---	---	5	144	36	2.8	481	7,400	.10	.22	.4	22
	Blackeye peas, immature seeds, cooked and drained:																	
585	From raw— 1 cup — 165	72	180	13	1	---	---	---	30	40	241	3.5	625	580	.50	.18	2.3	28
586	From frozen— 1 cup — 170	66	220	15	1	---	---	---	40	43	286	4.8	573	290	.68	.19	2.4	15
	Broccoli, cooked, drained:																	
	From raw:																	
587	Stalk, medium size— 1 stalk — 180	91	45	6	1	---	---	---	8	158	112	1.4	481	4,500	.16	.36	1.4	162
588	Stalks cut into 1/2-in pieces— 1 cup — 155	91	40	5	Trace	---	---	---	7	136	96	1.2	414	3,880	.14	.31	1.2	140
	From frozen:																	
589	Stalk, 4 1/2 to 5 in long— 1 stalk — 30	91	10	1	Trace	---	---	---	1	12	17	.2	66	570	.02	.03	.2	22
590	Chopped— 1 cup — 185	92	50	5	1	---	---	---	9	100	104	1.3	392	4,810	.11	.22	.9	105
591	**Brussels sprouts, cooked, drained:** From raw, 7-8 sprouts (1 1/4- to 1 1/2-in diam.). 1 cup — 155	88	55	7	1	---	---	---	10	50	112	1.7	423	810	.12	.22	1.2	135
592	From frozen— 1 cup — 155	89	50	5	Trace	---	---	---	10	33	95	1.2	457	880	.12	.16	.9	126

(B) VEGETABLE AND VEGETABLE PRODUCTS—Con.	(C) Grams	Per cent	(D) Cal-ories	(E) Grams	(F) Grams	(G) Grams	(H) Grams	(I) Grams	(J) Grams	(K) Milli-grams	(L) Milli-grams	(M) Milli-grams	(N) Milli-grams	(O) Inter-national units	(P) Milli-grams	(Q) Milli-grams	(R) Milli-grams	(S) Milli-grams
Cabbage:																		
Common varieties:																		
Raw:																		
593 Coarsely shredded or sliced-- 1 cup	70	92	15	1	Trace	---	---	---	4	34	20	0.3	163	90	0.04	0.04	0.02	33
594 Finely shredded or chopped-- 1 cup	90	92	20	1	Trace	---	---	---	5	44	26	.4	210	120	.05	.05	.3	42
595 Cooked, drained-- 1 cup	145	94	30	2	Trace	---	---	---	6	64	29	.4	236	190	.06	.06	.4	48
596 Red, coarsely shredded or sliced, 1 cup	70	90	20	1	Trace	---	---	---	5	29	25	.6	188	30	.06	.06	.3	43
597 Savoy, raw, coarsely shredded or sliced. 1 cup	70	92	15	2	Trace	---	---	---	3	47	38	.6	188	140	.04	.06	.2	39
598 Cabbage, celery (also called pe-tsai or wongbok), raw, 1-in pieces. 1 cup	75	95	10	1	Trace	---	---	---	2	32	30	.5	190	110	.04	.03	.5	19
599 Cabbage, white mustard (also called bokchoy or pakchoy), cooked, drained. 1 cup	170	95	25	2	Trace	---	---	---	4	252	56	1.0	364	5,270	.07	.14	1.2	26
Carrots:																		
Raw, without crowns and tips, scraped:																		
600 Whole, 7 1/2 by 1 1/8 in, or strips, 2 1/2 to 3 in long. 1 carrot or 18 strips ---	72	88	30	1	Trace	---	---	---	7	27	26	.5	246	7,930	.04	.04	.4	6
601 Grated-- 1 cup	110	88	45	1	Trace	---	---	---	11	41	40	.8	375	12,100	.07	.06	.7	9
602 Cooked (crosswise cuts), drained 1 cup	155	91	50	1	Trace	---	---	---	11	51	48	.9	344	16,280	.08	.08	.8	9
Canned:																		
603 Sliced, drained solids-- 1 cup	155	91	45	1	Trace	---	---	---	10	47	34	1.1	186	23,250	.03	.05	.6	3
604 Strained or junior (baby food)-- 1 oz (1 3/4 to 2 tbsp)--	28	92	10	Trace	Trace	---	---	---	2	7	6	.1	51	3,690	.01	.01	.1	1
Cauliflower:																		
605 Raw, chopped-- 1 cup	115	91	31	3	Trace	---	---	---	6	29	64	1.3	339	70	.13	.12	.8	90
Cooked, drained:																		
606 From raw (flower buds)-- 1 cup	125	93	30	3	Trace	---	---	---	5	26	53	.9	258	80	.11	.10	.8	69
607 From frozen (flowerets)-- 1 cup	180	94	30	3	Trace	---	---	---	6	31	68	.9	373	50	.07	.09	.7	74
608 Celery, Pascal type, raw: Stalk, large outer, 8 by 1 1/2 in, at root end. 1 stalk	40	94	5	Trace	Trace	---	---	---	2	16	11	.1	136	110	.01	.01	.1	4
609 Pieces, diced-- 1 cup	120	94	20	1	Trace	---	---	---	5	47	34	.4	409	320	.04	.04	.4	11
Collards, cooked, drained:																		
610 From raw (leaves without stems)-- 1 cup	190	90	65	7	1	---	---	---	10	357	99	1.5	498	14,820	.21	.38	2.3	144
611 From frozen (chopped)-- 1 cup	170	90	50	5	1	---	---	---	10	299	87	1.7	401	11,560	.10	.24	1.0	56
Corn, sweet:																		
Cooked, drained:																		
612 From raw, ear 5 by 1 3/4 in-- 1 ear[1]	140	74	70	2	1	---	---	---	16	2	69	.5	151	[62]310	.09	.08	1.1	7
From frozen:																		
613 Ear, 5 in long-- 1 ear[1]	229	73	120	4	1	---	---	---	27	4	121	1.0	291	[62]440	.18	.10	2.1	9
614 Kernels-- 1 cup	165	77	130	5	1	---	---	---	31	5	120	1.3	304	[62]580	.15	.10	2.5	8
Canned:																		
615 Cream style-- 1 cup	256	76	210	5	2	---	---	---	51	8	143	1.5	248	[62]840	.08	.13	2.6	13
Whole kernel:																		
616 Vacuum pack-- 1 cup	210	76	175	5	1	---	---	---	43	6	153	1.1	204	[62]740	.06	.13	2.3	7
617 Wet pack, drained solids-- 1 cup	165	76	140	4	1	---	---	---	33	8	81	.8	160	[62]580	.05	.08	1.5	7
Cowpeas. See Blackeye peas. (Items 585-586).																		
Cucumber slices, 1/8 in thick (large, 2 1/8-in diam.; small, 1 3/4-in diam.):																		
618 With peel-- 6 large or 8 small slices	28	95	5	Trace	Trace	---	---	---	1	7	8	.3	45	70	.01	.01	.1	3

(A)	(B)	(C)	(D)	(E)	(F)	(G)	(H)	(I)	(J)	(K)	(L)	(M)	(N)	(O)	(P)	(Q)	(R)	(S)	(T)
619	Without peel -- 6 1/2 large or 9 small pieces	28	96	5	Trace	Trace	—	—	—	1	7	5	0.1	45	Trace	.01	.01	0.1	3
620	Dandelion greens, cooked, drained -- 1 cup	105	90	35	2	Trace	—	—	—	7	147	44	1.9	244	12,290	.14	.17	1.6	19
621	Endive, curly (including escarole), raw, small pieces -- 1 cup	50	93	10	1	Trace	—	—	—	2	41	27	.9	147	1,650	.04	.07	.4	5
	Kale, cooked, drained:																		
622	From raw (leaves without stems and midribs) -- 1 cup	110	88	45	5	Trace	—	—	—	7	206	64	1.8	243	9,130	.11	.20	1.8	102
623	From frozen (leaf style) -- 1 cup	130	91	40	4	Trace	—	—	—	7	157	62	1.3	251	10,660	.08	.20	.9	49
	Lettuce, raw:																			
	Butterhead, as Boston types:																			
624	Head, 5-in diam -- 1 head[3]	220	95	25	2	Trace	—	—	—	4	57	42	3.3	430	1,580	.10	.10	.5	13
625	Leaves -- 1 outer or 2 inner or 3 heart leaves	15	95	Trace	Trace	Trace	—	—	—	Trace	5	4	.3	40	150	.01	.01	Trace	1
	Crisphead, as Iceberg:																			
626	Head, 6-in diam -- 1 head[4]	567	96	70	5	Trace	—	—	—	16	108	118	2.7	943	1,780	.32	.32	1.6	32
627	Wedge, 1/4 of head -- 1 wedge	135	96	20	1	Trace	—	—	—	4	27	30	.7	236	450	.08	.08	.4	8
628	Pieces, chopped or shredded -- 1 cup	55	96	5	Trace	Trace	—	—	—	2	11	12	.3	96	180	.03	.03	.2	3
629	Looseleaf (bunching varieties including romaine or cos), chopped or shredded pieces -- 1 cup	55	94	10	1	Trace	—	—	—	2	37	14	.8	145	1,050	.03	.04	.2	10
630	Mushrooms, raw, sliced or chopped -- 1 cup	70	90	20	2	Trace	—	—	—	3	4	81	.6	290	Trace	.07	.32	2.9	2
631	Mustard greens, without stems and midribs, cooked, drained -- 1 cup	140	93	30	3	Trace	—	—	—	6	193	45	2.5	308	8,120	.11	.20	.8	67
632	Okra pods, 3 by 5/8 in, cooked -- 10 pods	106	91	30	2	Trace	—	—	—	6	98	43	.5	184	520	.14	.19	1.0	21
	Onions:																			
	Mature:																			
	Raw:																			
633	Chopped -- 1 cup	170	89	65	3	Trace	—	—	—	15	46	61	.9	267	Trace[5]	.05	.07	.3	17
634	Sliced -- 1 cup	115	89	45	2	Trace	—	—	—	10	31	41	.6	181	Trace[5]	.03	.05	.2	12
635	Cooked (whole or sliced), drained -- 1 cup	210	92	60	3	Trace	—	—	—	14	50	61	.8	231	Trace[5]	.06	.06	.4	15
636	Young green, bulb (3/8 in diam.) and white portion of top -- 6 onions	30	88	15	Trace	Trace	—	—	—	3	12	12	.2	69	Trace	.02	.01	.1	8
637	Parsley, raw, chopped -- 1 tbsp	4	85	Trace	Trace	Trace	—	—	—	Trace	7	2	.2	25	300	Trace	.01	Trace	6
638	Parsnips, cooked (diced or 2-in lengths) -- 1 cup	155	82	100	2	1	—	—	—	23	70	96	.9	587	50	.11	.12	.2	16
	Peas, green:																			
	Canned:																			
639	Whole, drained solids -- 1 cup	170	77	150	8	1	—	—	—	29	44	129	3.2	163	1,170	.15	.10	1.4	14
640	Strained (baby food) -- 1 oz (1 3/4 to 2 tbsp)	28	86	15	1	Trace	—	—	—	3	3	18	.3	28	140	.02	.03	.3	3
641	Frozen, cooked, drained -- 1 cup	160	82	110	8	Trace	—	—	—	19	30	138	3.0	216	960	.43	.14	2.7	21
642	Peppers, hot, red, without seeds, dried (ground chili powder, added seasonings) -- 1 tsp	2	9	5	Trace	Trace	—	—	—	1	5	4	.3	20	1,300	Trace	.02	.2	Trace
	Peppers, sweet (about 5 per lb, whole), stem and seeds removed:																			
643	Raw -- 1 pod	74	93	15	1	Trace	—	—	—	4	7	16	.5	157	310	.06	.06	.4	94
644	Cooked, boiled, drained -- 1 pod	73	95	15	1	Trace	—	—	—	3	7	12	.4	109	310	.05	.05	.3	70
	Potatoes, cooked:																			
645	Baked, peeled after baking (about 2 per lb, raw) -- 1 potato	156	75	145	4	Trace	—	—	—	33	14	101	1.1	782	Trace	.15	.07	2.7	31
	Boiled (about 3 per lb, raw):																			
646	Peeled after boiling -- 1 potato	137	80	105	3	Trace	—	—	—	23	10	72	.8	556	Trace	.12	.05	2.0	22
647	Peeled before boiling -- 1 potato	135	83	90	3	Trace	—	—	—	20	8	57	.7	385	Trace	.12	.05	1.6	22
	French-fried, strip, 2 to 3 1/2 in long:																			
648	Prepared from raw -- 10 strips	50	45	135	2	7	1.7	1.2	3.3	18	8	56	.7	427	Trace	.07	.04	1.6	11
649	Frozen, oven heated -- 10 strips	50	53	110	2	4	1.1	.8	2.1	17	5	43	.9	326	Trace	.07	.01	1.3	11
650	Hashed brown, prepared from frozen -- 1 cup	155	56	345	3	18	4.6	3.2	9.0	45	28	78	1.9	439	Trace	.11	.03	1.6	12
	Mashed, prepared from—																			
	Raw:																			
651	Milk added -- 1 cup	210	83	135	4	1	.7	.4	Trace	27	50	103	.8	548	40	.17	.11	2.1	21

[1] Weight includes cob. Without cob, weight is 77 g for item 612, 126 g for item 613.
[2] Based on yellow varieties. For white varieties, value is trace.
[3] Weight includes refuse of outer leaves and core. Without these parts, weight is 163 g.
[4] Weight includes core. Without core, weight is 539 g.
[5] Value based on white-fleshed varieties. For yellow-fleshed varieties, value in International Units (I.U.) is 70 for item 633, 50 for item 634, and 80 for item 635.

MISCELLANEOUS ITEMS

(A)	(B)	(C)	(D)	(E)	(F)	(G)	(H)	(I)	(J)	(K)	(L)	(M)	(N)	(O)	(P)	(Q)	(R)	(S)
	Baking powders for home use:																	
	Sodium aluminum sulfate:																	
681	With monocalcium phosphate monohydrate----- 1 tsp----- 3.0	2	5	Trace	Trace	0	0	0	1	58	87	--	5	0	0	0	0	0
682	With monocalcium phosphate monohydrate, calcium sulfate----- 1 tsp----- 2.9	1	5	Trace	Trace	0	0	0	1	183	45	--		0	0	0	0	0
683	Straight phosphate----- 1 tsp----- 3.8	2	5	Trace	Trace	0	0	0	1	239	359	--	6	0	0	0	0	0
684	Low sodium----- 1 tsp----- 4.3	2	5	Trace	Trace	0	0	0	2	207	314	--	471	0	0	0	0	0
685	Barbecue sauce----- 1 cup----- 250	81	230	4	17	2.2	4.3	10.0	20	53	50	2.0	435	900	.03	.03	.8	13
	Beverages, alcoholic:																	
686	Beer----- 12 fl oz----- 360	92	150	1	0	0	0	0	14	18	108	Trace	90	--	.01	.11	2.2	--
	Gin, rum, vodka, whisky:																	
687	80-proof----- 1 1/2-fl oz jigger----- 42	67	95			0	0	0	Trace	--	--	--	--	--	--	--	--	--
688	90-proof----- 1 1/2-fl oz jigger----- 42	64	105			0	0	0	Trace	--	--	--	--	--	--	--	--	--
689	100-proof----- 1 1/2-fl oz jigger----- 42	62	110			0	0	0	Trace	--	--	--	--	--	--	--	--	--
	Wines:																	
690	Dessert----- 3 1/2-fl oz glass----- 103	77	140	Trace	0	0	0	0	8	8	10	.4	77	--	.01	.02	.2	--
691	Table----- 3 1/2-fl oz glass----- 102	86	85	Trace	0	0	0	0	4	9			94	--	Trace	.01	.1	--
	Beverages, carbonated, sweetened, nonalcoholic:																	
692	Carbonated water----- 12 fl oz----- 366	92	115	0	0	0	0	0	29	--	--	--	--	--	0	0	0	0
693	Cola type----- 12 fl oz----- 369	90	145	0	0	0	0	0	37	--	--	--	--	--	0	0	0	0
694	Fruit-flavored sodas and Tom Collins mixer----- 12 fl oz----- 372	88	170	0	0	0	0	0	45	--	--	--	--	--	0	0	0	0
695	Ginger ale----- 12 fl oz----- 366	92	115	0	0	0	0	0	29	--	--	--	0	--	0	0	0	0
696	Root beer----- 12 fl oz----- 370	90	150	0	0	0	0	0	39	--	--	--	0	--	0	0	0	0
	Chili powder. See Peppers, hot, red (item 642).																	
	Chocolate:																	
697	Bitter or baking----- 1 oz----- 28	2	145	3	15	8.9	4.9	.4	8	22	109	1.9	235	20	.01	.07	.4	0
	Semisweet. See Candy, chocolate (item 539).																	
698	Gelatin, dry----- 1 7-g envelope----- 7	13	25	6	Trace	0	0	0	0	--	--	--	--	--	--	--	--	--
699	Gelatin dessert prepared with gelatin dessert powder and water----- 1 cup----- 240	84	140	4	0	0	0	0	34	--	--	--	--	--	--	--	--	--
700	Mustard, prepared, yellow----- 1 tsp or individual serving pouch or cup----- 5	80	5	Trace	Trace	--	--	--	Trace	4	4	.1	7	--	--	--	--	--
	Olives, pickled, canned:																	
701	Green----- 4 medium or 3 extra large or 2 giant----- 16	78	15	Trace	2	.2	1.2	.1	Trace	8	2	.2	7	40	Trace	Trace	--	--
702	Ripe, Mission----- 3 small or 2 large----- 10	73	15	Trace	2	.2	1.2	.1	Trace	9	1	.1	2	10	Trace	Trace	--	--
	Pickles, cucumber:																	
703	Dill, medium, whole, 3 3/4 in long, 1 1/4-in diam----- 1 pickle----- 65	93	5	Trace	Trace			Trace	17	17	14	.7	130	70	Trace	.01	Trace	4
704	Fresh-pack, slices 1 1/2-in diam, 1/4 in thick----- 2 slices----- 15	79	10	Trace	Trace				3	5	4	.3	--	20	Trace	Trace	Trace	1
705	Sweet, gherkin, small, whole, about 2 1/2 in long, 3/4-in diam----- 1 pickle----- 15	61	20	Trace	Trace				5	2	2	.2	--	10	Trace	Trace	Trace	1
706	Relish, finely chopped, sweet----- 1 tbsp----- 15	63	20	Trace	Trace				5	3	2	.1		--	0	0	0	0
	Popcorn. See items 476-478.																	
707	Popsicle, 3-fl oz size----- 1 popsicle----- 95	80	70	0	0	0	0	0	18	0	--	Trace	--	0	0	0	0	0

*Weight includes cores and stem ends. Without these parts, weight is 123 g.

**Based on year-round average. For tomatoes marketed from November through May, value is about 12 mg; from June through October, 32 mg.

***Applies to product without calcium salts added. Value for products with calcium salts added may be as much as 63 mg for whole tomatoes, 241 mg for cut forms.

****Weight includes pits. Without pits, weight is 13 g for item 701, 9 g for item 702.

MISCELLANEOUS ITEMS—Con.

(A)	(B)	Grams	(C) Per cent	(D) Calories	(E) Grams	(F) Grams	(G) Grams	(H) Grams	(I) Grams	(J) Grams	(K) Milligrams	(L) Milligrams	(M) Milligrams	(N) Milligrams	(O) International units	(P) Milligrams	(Q) Milligrams	(R) Milligrams	(S) Milligrams
	Soups:																		
	Canned, condensed:																		
	Prepared with equal volume of milk:																		
708	Cream of chicken——— 1 cup	245	85	180	7	10	4.2	3.6	1.3	15	172	152	0.5	260	610	0.05	0.27	0.7	2
709	Cream of mushroom— 1 cup	245	83	215	7	14	5.4	2.9	4.6	16	191	169	.5	279	250	.05	.34	.7	1
710	Tomato———— 1 cup	250	84	175	7	7	3.4	1.7	1.0	23	168	155	.8	418	1,200	.10	.25	1.3	15
	Prepared with equal volume of water:																		
711	Bean with pork——— 1 cup	250	84	170	8	6	1.2	1.8	2.4	22	63	128	2.3	395	650	.13	.08	1.0	3
712	Beef broth, bouillon, consomme. 1 cup	240	96	30	5	0	0	0	0	3	Trace	31	.5	130	Trace	Trace	.02	1.2	
713	Beef noodle——— 1 cup	240	93	65	4	3	.6	.7	.8	7	7	48	1.0	77	50	.05	.07	1.0	Trace
714	Clam chowder, Manhattan type (with tomatoes, without milk). 1 cup	245	92	80	2	3	.5	.4	1.3	12	34	47	1.0	184	880	.02	.02	1.0	
715	Cream of chicken——— 1 cup	240	92	95	3	6	1.6	2.3	1.1	8	24	34	.5	79	410	.02	.05	.5	Trace
716	Cream of mushroom—— 1 cup	240	90	135	2	10	2.6	1.7	4.5	10	41	50	.5	98	70	.02	.12	.7	Trace
717	Minestrone——— 1 cup	245	90	105	5	3	.7	.9	1.3	14	37	59	1.0	314	2,350	.07	.05	1.0	
718	Split pea——— 1 cup	245	85	145	9	3	1.1	1.2	.4	21	29	149	1.5	270	440	.25	.15	1.5	1
719	Tomato——— 1 cup	245	91	90	2	3	.5	.5	1.0	16	15	34	.7	230	1,000	.05	.05	1.2	12
720	Vegetable beef——— 1 cup	245	92	80	5	2				10	12	49	.7	162	2,700	.05	.05	1.0	
721	Vegetarian——— 1 cup	245	92	80	2	2				13	20	39	1.0	172	2,940	.05	.05	1.0	
	Dehydrated:																		
722	Bouillon cube, 1/2 in—— 1 cube	4	4	5	1	Trace				Trace				4					
	Mixes: Unprepared:																		
723	Onion——— 1 1/2-oz pkg	43	3	150	6	5	1.1	2.3	1.0	23	42	49	.6	238	30	.05	.03	.3	6
	Prepared with water:																		
724	Chicken noodle——— 1 cup	240	95	55	2	1				8	7	19	.2	19	50	.07	.05	.5	Trace
725	Onion——— 1 cup	240	96	35	1	1				6	10	12	.2	58	Trace	Trace	Trace	.5	2
726	Tomato vegetable with noodles. 1 cup	240	93	65	1	1				12	7	19	.2	29	480	.05	.02	.5	5
727	Vinegar, cider——— 1 tbsp	15	94	Trace	Trace	0	0	0	0	1	1	1	.1	15					
728	White sauce, medium, with enriched flour. 1 cup	250	73	405	10	31	19.3	7.8	.8	22	288	233	.5	348	1,150	.12	.43	.7	2
	Yeast:																		
729	Baker's, dry, active—— 1 pkg	7	5	20	3	Trace				3	3	90	1.1	140	Trace	.16	.38	2.6	Trace
730	Brewer's, dry——— 1 tbsp	8	5	25	3	Trace				3	[1]17	140	1.4	152	Trace	1.25	.34	3.0	Trace

[1]Value may vary from 6 to 60 mg.

APPENDIX G.

RECOMMENDED DAILY DIETARY ALLOWANCES (RDA)

(Designed for the maintenance of good nutrition of practically all healthy persons in the United States.)

Sex-age category	Age (Years) From	To	Weight Kilograms	Pounds	Height Centimeters	Inches	Food energy Calories	Protein Grams	Minerals Calcium Milligrams	Phosphorus Milligrams	Iron Milligrams	Vitamin A International units	Thiamin Milligrams	Riboflavin Milligrams	Niacin Milligrams	Ascorbic acid Milligrams
Infants …	0	0.5	6	14	60	24	kg x 117 / lb x 53.2	kg x 2.2 / lb x 1.0	360	240	10	1,400	0.3	0.4	5	35
	0.5	1	9	20	71	28	kg x 108 / lb x 49.1	kg x 2.0 / lb x 0.9	540	400	15	2,000	.5	.6	8	35
Children …	1	3	13	28	86	34	1,300	23	800	800	15	2,000	.7	.8	9	40
	4	6	20	44	110	44	1,800	30	800	800	10	2,500	.9	1.1	12	40
	7	10	30	66	135	54	2,400	36	800	800	10	3,300	1.2	1.2	16	40
Males ……	11	14	44	97	158	63	2,800	44	1,200	1,200	18	5,000	1.4	1.5	18	45
	15	18	61	134	172	69	3,000	54	1,200	1,200	18	5,000	1.5	1.8	20	45
	19	22	67	147	172	69	3,000	54	800	800	10	5,000	1.5	1.8	20	45
	23	50	70	154	172	69	2,700	56	800	800	10	5,000	1.4	1.6	18	45
	51+		70	154	172	69	2,400	56	800	800	10	5,000	1.2	1.5	16	45
Females …	11	14	44	97	155	62	2,400	44	1,200	1,200	18	4,000	1.2	1.3	16	45
	15	18	54	119	162	65	2,100	48	1,200	1,200	18	4,000	1.1	1.4	14	45
	19	22	58	128	162	65	2,100	46	800	800	18	4,000	1.1	1.4	14	45
	23	50	58	128	162	65	2,000	46	800	800	18	4,000	1.0	1.2	13	45
	51+		58	128	162	65	1,800	46	800	800	10	4,000	1.0	1.2	12	45
Pregnant							+300	+30	1,200	1,200	[2]+18	5,000	+ .3	+ .3	+2	60
Lactating							+500	+20	1,200	1,200	18	6,000	+ .3	+ .5	+4	80

APPENDIX H. XBX EXERCISE PLAN
(RCAF 10 Basic Exercises For Fitness)

THE PLAN

The RCAF (Royal Canadian Air Force) XBX plan for fitness provides a series of exercises, explains where to start, and indicates how fast and how far you should progress to achieve a desirable level of physical fitness. The program is designed to require only 12 minutes a day, no equipment and very little space.

The XBX plan is composed of four charts of ten exercises which are arranged in progressive order of difficulty. The charts are divided into 48 levels — 12 in each chart. The time limit for each exercise on all charts remains the same, but the number of times the exercise is performed within the time limit is increased at each level within each chart. As you move from one chart to the next higher one, the exercises are modified to become more difficult.

PROCEDURE

Select your goal according to your age and the recommended minimum number of days at each level by using the table below:

If Your Age is	Your Goal is Level	Recommended Minimum Number of Days at Each Level on			
		Chart I	Chart II	Chart III	Chart IV
7- 8 years	30	1	1	2	x
9-10 years	34	1	1	2	x
11-12 years	38	1	1	2	3
13-14 years	41	1	1	2	3
15-17 years	44	1	1	2	3
18-19 years	40	1	2	3	4
20-25 years	35	1	2	3	x
26-30 years	30	2	3	5	x
31-35 years	26	2	4	6	x
36-40 years	22	4	6	x	x
41-45 years	19	5	7	x	x
46-50 years	16	7	8	x	x
51-55 years	11	8	x	x	x

Start at Level I on Chart I and then continue through the levels and charts until you reach the goal level recommended for you or until you feel you are exercising at your maximum capacity. When you have reached your goal you should require only 3 exercise periods a week to maintain it.

NOTE: Based on the Royal Canadian Air Force Exercise Plan for Physical Fitness, and adaptations of exercises from *Body Mechanics* by Lindsey, Jones and Whitley.

		EXERCISE									
		1	2	3	4	5	6	7	8	9	10
	12	9	8	10	40	26	20	28	14	14".·	170
	11	9	8	10	40	24	18	26	13	14	160
	10	9	8	10	40	22	16	25	12	12	150
L	9	7	7	8	36	20	14	23	10	11	140
E	8	7	7	8	36	18	12	20	9	10	125
V	7	7	7	8	36	16	12	18	8	10	115
E	6	5	5	7	28	14	10	16	7	8	100
L	5	5	5	7	28	12	8	13	6	6	90
	4	5	5	7	28	10	8	10	5	6	80
	3	3	4	5	24	8	6	8	4	4	70
	2	3	4	5	24	6	4	6	3	3	60
	1	3	4	5	24	4	4	4	3	2	50
Minutes for each Exercise		2				2	1	1	2	1	3

PHASE I EXERCISES—

1.a. **Toe Touch.** Feet 12″ apart; arms overhead; try to touch floor.

b. **Alternate.*** Same as above, except perform in sitting position.

2. **Knee Raise.** Raise alternate knees and pull toward chest with arms; keep back straight; left plus right is 1 count.

3. **Lateral Bend.** Feet 12″ apart; alternate sideward, bending to right and left, sliding hand down leg as far as possible; left plus right is 1 count.

4. **Arm Circle.*** Feet 12″ apart; make large backward circles with one arm; half repetitions with left arm, half with right.

5. **Partial Sit-ups.** Back lying; arms at side; raise head and shoulders until you can see your heels.

6.a. **Chest and Leg Raise.** Front lying; hands under thighs; raise head and shoulders and alternate legs as high as possible; left is one count, right is one count.

b. **Knee-to-Nose Touch.*** (For those with lordosis.) On hands and knees, try to touch nose with knee; then extend leg backward *parallel* with floor while raising head; do not arch back; half of repetitions with right leg, half with left.

7. **Side Leg Raise.** Side lying; use arms for balance; raise upper leg 18-24 inches; half of repetitions left leg, half right.

8. **Push-ups.** Front lying; hands under shoulders; push up and rock back on heels; keep hands and knees on floor; return to starting position.

9. **Leg Lift.** Back lying; arms at side; raise alternate legs perpendicular to floor; left plus right is 1 count.

10. **Run and Hop.** Run in place; lift knees and feet at least 4″ high; left plus right is 1 count; after 50 counts, jump up and down 10 times, lifting feet at least 4″ high.

  ° Starred exercises are those revised by the authors.
  Those persons with lordosis should perform exercise 6.b. rather than 6.a.

PHASE II

		EXERCISE									
		1	2	3	4	5	6	7	8	9	10
	24	15	16	12	30	35	38	50	28	20	210
	23	15	16	12	30	33	36	48	26	18	200
	22	15	16	12	30	31	34	48	24	18	200
L	21	13	14	11	26	29	32	44	23	16	190
E	20	13	14	11	26	27	31	42	21	16	175
V	19	13	14	11	26	24	29	40	20	14	160
E	18	12	12	9	20	22	27	38	18	14	150
L	17	12	12	9	20	19	24	36	16	12	150
	16	12	12	9	20	16	21	34	14	10	140
	15	10	10	7	18	14	18	32	14	10	130
	14	10	10	7	18	11	15	30	10	8	120
	13	10	10	7	18	9	12	28	8	8	120
Minutes for each Exercise		2				2	1	1	2	1	3

PHASE II

PHASE II EXERCISES—(Same as Phase I, except at noted.)
1. **Toe Touch.** Bob once, touching floor a second time.
2. **Knee Raise.**
3. **Lateral Bend.** Bob once, sliding hand down leg a second time.
4. **Arm Circle.°** Circle both arms backward simultaneously.
5. **Rocking Sit-ups.** Back lying with knees bent; arms overhead; swing arms and sit up while legs extend; try to touch toes; return to starting position.
6.a. **Chest and Leg Raise.** Lift head and shoulders and both legs at same time.
   b. **Knee-to-Nose Touch.°**
7. **Side Leg Raise.** Try to raise leg perpendicular to floor.
8. **Knee Push-ups.** Keep body line straight while pushing up and down; do not rock back on heels.
9. **Leg Overs.** Back lying; arms out at shoulder level; raise one leg to perpendicular and try to touch opposite hand with toes; return to perpendicular and to starting position; alternate legs; left is 1 count; right is 1 count.
10. **Run-and-Stride Jump.** Do 10 jumping-jacks after every 50 runs.

° Starred exercises are those revised by the authors.
Those persons with lordosis should perform exercise 6.b. rather than 6.a.

PHASE III

		EXERCISE									
		1	2	3	4	5	6	7	8	9	10
	36	15	22	18	40	42	40	60	40	20	240
	35	15	22	18	40	41	39	60	39	20	230
L	34	15	22	18	40	40	38	58	37	19	220
	33	13	20	16	36	39	36	58	35	19	210
E	32	13	20	16	36	37	36	56	34	18	200
	31	13	20	16	36	35	34	56	32	16	200
V	30	12	18	14	30	33	33	54	30	15	190
	29	12	18	14	30	32	31	54	29	14	180
E	28	12	18	14	30	31	30	52	27	12	170
	27	10	16	12	24	29	30	52	25	11	160
L	26	10	16	12	24	27	29	50	23	9	150
	25	10	16	12	24	26	28	48	22	8	140
Minutes for each Exercise		2				2	1	1	2	1	3

PHASE III

PHASE III EXERCISES—(Same as Phase II, except as noted.)
1. **Toe Touch.** Feet 16" apart; arms overhead; bob, and touch floor to left, center, and right.
2. **Knee Raise.**
3. **Lateral Bend.** Raise one arm overhead with elbow bent; bend and reach to opposite side; alternate sides.
4. **Arm Circle.°** Alternate arms backward like a windmill; left plus right is 1 count.
5. **Sit-ups.** Keep legs straight; start with arms at sides.
6.a. **Chest and Leg Raise.** Arms stretched sideward at shoulder level; lift arms, head, shoulders, and both legs simultaneously.
   b. **Knee-to-Nose Touch.°**
7. **Side Leg Raise.**
8. **Elbow Push-ups.°** Front lying; elbows under shoulders; forearms on floor with hands clasped; raise hips from floor until body line is straight and supported by forearms and toes; rock forward and backward from toes, bringing upper arms near forearms; keep back straight.
9. **Legs-Over Tuck.** Back lying; bend knees to chest; keep shoulders on floor and roll, touching tucked knees to floor on left, then right for 1 count; keep knees together and near chest throughout; return to starting position.
10. **Run and Half-Knee Bends.** After 50 runs raising feet 6" high, do 10 half-knee bends with hands on hips; 90-110° angle of knee flexion.

° Starred exercises are those revised by the authors.
Those persons with lordosis should perform exercise 6.b. rather than 6.a.

PHASE IV

		EXERCISE									
		1	2	3	4	5	6	7	8	9	10
	48	15	26	15	32	48	46	58	30	16	230
	47	15	26	15	32	45	45	56	27	15	220
	46	15	26	15	32	44	44	54	24	14	210
L	45	13	24	14	30	42	43	52	21	13	200
E	44	13	24	14	30	40	42	50	19	13	190
V	43	13	24	14	30	38	40	48	16	12	175
E	42	12	22	12	28	35	39	46	13	10	160
L	41	12	22	12	28	32	38	44	11	9	150
	40	12	22	12	28	30	38	40	9	8	140
	39	10	20	10	26	29	36	38	8	7	130
	38	10	20	10	26	27	35	36	7	6	115
	37	10	20	10	26	25	34	34	6	5	100
Minutes for each Exercise				2			2	1	1	2	1	3

PHASE IV

PHASE IV EXERCISES—(Same as Phase III, except as noted.)

1. **Toe Touch.** Bob left, center, right.
2. **Knee Raise.**
3. **Lateral Bend.** Arm overhead; bob a second time to each side.
4. **Arm Fling.** Feet 12" apart; elbows up and out; finger tips touching in front of chest; jerk elbows back and return to start; fling arms back as far as possible, straightening elbow; keep the jerk and fling high; each fling counts 1.
5. **Sit-ups.** Legs straight; hands clasped behind neck; keep feet on floor, holding them down if necessary.
6.a. **Chest and Leg Raise.** Hands clasped behind neck.
   b. **Knee-to-Nose Touch.**°
7. **Side Leg Raise.** Right side toward floor; weight supported on right hand (arm straight) and side of right foot; left arm for balance; *keep body line straight* and raise left leg parallel to floor; half of repetitions on right side, half on left.
8. **Push-ups.** Body line straight from shoulders to toes; do push-ups from toes touching chest each time.
9. **Legs-Over Straight.**° Bend both knees to chest, then raise legs perpendicular to floor; keep shoulders on floor and roll, trying to touch feet to hand on each side; return to perpendicular, then starting position; left plus right is 1 count.
10. **Run and Semi-Squat Jump.** After each 50 runs, do 10 semi-squat jumps by half crouching, with hands on knees, arm straight; one foot slightly ahead of other; jump so feet leave floor and body is erect; land with feet in reverse position.

° Starred exercises are those revised by the authors.
Those persons with lordosis should perform exercise 6.b. rather than 6.a.

NOTE: Based on the "Royal Canadian Air Force Exercise Plan for Physical Fitness" and adaptations of exercises from "Body Mechanics" by Lindsey, Jones, & Whitley.

APPENDIX I. CIRCUIT TRAINING PROGRAM

An excellent method of developing many phases of fitness is circuit training. A circuit usually consists of 7-12 stations at which each exercise is done for a specified number of times. Activities at the stations can include those for strength, muscular endurance, flexibility, power, or cardiovascular endurance. There are various ways of setting up a circuit which follows the principle of progressive overload:

1. Attempting to complete the circuit in as little time as possible.

2. Increasing the number of repetitions at each station within the same time period.

3. Completing the circuit as many times as possible within a set time.

Suggested exercises to be included in a circuit are:

1. Squat Thrusts

2. Curls or Sit-Ups

3. Push-Ups

4. V Sit-Ups

5. Bench Stepping

6. Run in Place

7. Jumping Jacks

8. Alternate Toe Touch

9. Sprinter

10. Rope Skipping

11. Leg Raises and Kicks (flutter or scissor)

Another variation to the usual circuit is to have students run one lap around all the stations before moving to the next designated station. This adds significantly to the cardiovascular benefits of the program.

APPENDIX J. CALORIC EXPENDITURE PER MINUTE FOR VARIOUS ACTIVITIES

Calorie Expenditure per Minute for Various Activities

Body Weight

Activity	90	99	108	117	125	134	143	152	161	170	178	187	196	205	213	222	231	240	249	257	266	275
Archery	3.1	3.4	3.7	4.0	4.3	4.6	4.9	5.2	5.5	5.8	6.1	6.4	6.7	7.0	7.3	7.6	7.9	8.2	8.5	8.8	9.1	9.4
Badminton (recreation)	3.4	3.8	4.1	4.4	4.8	5.1	5.4	5.6	6.1	6.4	6.8	7.1	7.4	7.8	8.1	8.3	8.8	9.1	9.4	9.8	10.1	10.4
Badminton (competition)	5.9	6.4	7.0	7.6	8.1	8.7	9.3	9.9	10.4	11.0	11.6	12.1	12.7	13.3	13.9	14.4	15.0	15.6	16.1	16.7	17.3	17.9
Baseball (player)	2.8	3.1	3.4	3.6	3.9	4.2	4.5	4.7	5.0	5.3	5.5	5.8	6.1	6.4	6.6	6.9	7.2	7.5	7.7	8.0	8.3	8.6
Baseball (pitcher)	3.5	3.9	4.3	4.6	5.0	5.3	5.7	6.0	6.4	6.7	7.1	7.4	7.8	8.1	8.5	8.8	9.2	9.5	9.9	10.2	10.6	10.9
Basketball (half-court)	2.5	3.3	3.5	3.8	4.1	4.4	4.7	4.9	5.3	5.6	5.9	6.2	6.4	6.7	7.0	7.3	7.5	7.6	8.2	8.5	8.8	9.0
Basketball (moderate)	4.2	4.6	5.0	5.5	5.9	6.3	6.7	7.1	7.5	7.9	8.3	8.8	9.2	9.6	10.0	10.4	10.8	11.2	11.6	12.1	12.5	12.9
Basketball (competition)	5.9	6.5	7.1	7.7	8.2	8.8	9.4	10.0	10.6	11.1	11.7	12.3	12.9	13.5	14.0	14.6	15.0	15.6	16.3	16.9	17.5	18.1
Bicycling (level) 5.5 mph	3.0	3.3	3.6	3.9	4.2	4.5	4.8	5.1	5.4	5.6	5.9	6.2	6.5	6.8	7.1	7.4	7.7	8.0	8.3	8.6	8.9	9.2
Bicycling (level) 13 mph	6.4	7.1	7.7	8.3	8.9	9.6	10.2	10.8	11.4	12.1	12.7	13.4	14.0	14.6	15.2	15.9	16.5	17.1	17.8	18.4	19.0	19.6
Bowling (nonstop)	4.0	4.4	4.8	5.2	5.6	5.9	6.3	6.7	7.1	7.5	7.9	8.3	8.7	9.1	9.5	9.8	10.2	10.6	11.0	11.4	11.8	12.2
Boxing (sparring)	3.0	3.3	3.6	3.9	4.2	4.5	4.8	5.1	5.4	5.6	5.9	6.2	6.5	6.8	7.1	7.4	7.7	8.0	8.3	8.6	8.9	9.2
Calisthenics	3.0	3.3	3.6	3.9	4.2	4.5	4.8	5.1	5.4	5.6	5.9	6.2	6.5	6.8	7.1	7.4	7.7	8.0	8.3	8.6	8.9	9.2
Canoeing, 2.5 mph	1.8	1.9	2.0	2.2	2.3	2.5	2.7	3.0	3.2	3.4	3.6	3.7	3.9	4.1	4.4	4.6	4.7	4.8	5.0	5.1	5.3	5.5
Canoeing, 4.0 mph	4.2	4.6	5.0	5.5	5.9	6.3	6.7	7.1	7.5	7.9	8.3	8.7	9.2	9.4	10.0	10.5	10.8	11.2	11.6	12.0	12.4	12.9
Dance, modern (moderate)	2.5	2.8	3.0	3.2	3.5	3.7	4.0	4.2	4.5	4.7	5.0	5.2	5.4	5.7	5.9	6.2	6.4	6.7	6.9	7.2	7.4	7.6
Dance, modern (vigorous)	3.4	3.7	4.1	4.4	4.7	5.1	5.4	5.7	6.1	6.4	6.7	7.1	7.4	7.7	8.1	8.4	8.7	9.1	9.4	9.7	10.1	10.4
Dance, fox-trot	2.7	2.9	3.2	3.4	3.7	4.0	4.2	4.5	4.7	5.0	5.3	5.5	5.8	6.0	6.3	6.6	6.8	7.1	7.3	7.6	7.9	8.1
Dance, rumba	4.2	4.6	5.0	5.4	5.8	6.2	6.6	7.0	7.4	7.8	8.2	8.6	9.0	9.4	9.7	10.2	10.6	11.0	11.5	11.9	12.3	12.6
Dance, square	4.1	4.5	4.9	5.3	5.7	6.1	6.5	6.9	7.3	7.8	8.1	8.5	8.9	9.3	9.7	10.1	10.5	10.9	11.3	11.7	12.1	12.4
Dance, waltz	3.1	3.4	3.7	4.0	4.3	4.6	4.9	5.2	5.5	5.8	6.1	6.4	6.7	7.0	7.3	7.6	7.9	8.2	8.5	8.8	9.1	9.4
Fencing (moderate)	3.0	3.3	3.6	3.9	4.2	4.5	4.8	5.1	5.4	5.6	6.0	6.2	6.5	6.8	7.1	7.4	7.7	8.0	8.3	8.6	8.9	9.2
Fencing (vigorous)	6.2	6.8	7.4	8.0	8.6	9.2	9.8	10.4	11.0	11.6	12.2	12.8	13.4	14.0	14.6	15.2	15.8	16.4	17.0	17.6	18.2	18.8
Football (moderate)	3.0	3.3	3.6	4.0	4.2	4.5	4.8	5.1	5.4	5.7	6.0	6.2	6.5	6.8	7.1	7.4	7.7	8.0	8.3	8.6	8.9	9.2
Football (vigorous)	5.0	5.5	6.0	6.4	6.9	7.4	7.9	8.4	8.9	9.4	9.8	10.3	10.8	11.3	11.8	12.3	12.8	13.2	13.7	14.2	14.7	15.2
Golf, 2-some	3.3	3.6	3.9	4.2	4.5	4.8	5.2	5.5	5.8	6.1	6.4	6.7	7.1	7.4	7.7	8.0	8.3	8.6	9.0	9.3	9.6	10.0
Golf, 4-some	2.4	2.7	2.9	3.2	3.4	3.6	3.9	4.1	4.3	4.6	4.8	5.1	5.3	5.5	5.8	6.0	6.2	6.5	6.7	7.0	7.2	7.4
Handball	5.9	6.4	7.0	7.6	8.1	8.7	9.3	9.9	10.4	11.0	11.6	12.1	12.7	13.3	13.9	14.4	15.0	15.6	16.1	16.7	17.3	17.9
Hiking, 40 lb. pack, 3.0 mph	4.1	4.5	4.9	5.3	5.7	6.1	6.5	6.9	7.3	7.7	8.1	8.5	8.9	9.3	9.7	10.1	10.5	10.9	11.3	11.7	12.1	12.5
Horseback Riding (walk)	2.0	2.3	2.4	2.6	2.8	3.0	3.1	3.3	3.5	3.7	3.9	4.1	4.3	4.5	4.7	4.9	5.1	5.3	5.5	5.7	5.8	6.0
Horseback Riding (trot)	4.1	4.4	4.8	5.2	5.6	6.0	6.4	6.8	7.2	7.6	8.0	8.4	8.8	9.2	9.6	10.0	10.4	10.8	11.1	11.6	12.0	12.4
Horseshoe Pitching	2.1	2.3	2.5	2.7	3.0	3.3	3.4	3.6	3.8	4.0	4.2	4.4	4.6	4.8	5.0	5.2	5.4	5.6	5.8	6.0	6.3	6.5
Judo, Karate	7.7	8.5	9.2	10.0	10.7	11.5	12.2	13.0	13.7	14.5	15.2	16.0	16.7	17.5	18.2	19.0	19.7	20.5	21.2	22.0	22.7	23.5
Mountain Climbing	6.0	6.5	7.2	7.8	8.4	9.0	9.6	10.1	10.7	11.3	11.9	12.5	13.1	13.7	14.3	14.8	15.4	16.0	16.6	17.2	17.8	18.4
Paddleball, Racquetball	5.9	6.4	7.0	7.6	8.1	8.7	9.3	9.9	10.4	11.0	11.6	12.1	12.7	13.3	13.9	14.4	15.0	15.6	16.1	16.7	17.3	17.9
Pool, Billiards	1.1	1.2	1.3	1.4	1.5	1.6	1.7	1.8	1.9	2.0	2.1	2.2	2.4	2.5	2.6	2.7	2.8	2.9	3.0	3.1	3.2	3.3
Push Ups	4.3	4.7	5.1	5.6	6.0	6.4	6.8	7.2	7.7	8.1	8.5	8.9	9.4	9.8	10.2	10.6	11.0	11.5	11.9	12.3	12.7	13.2
Racquetball	6.0	6.6	7.2	7.8	8.3	8.9	9.5	10.1	10.7	11.3	11.9	12.5	13.1	13.7	14.2	14.8	15.4	16.0	16.6	17.2	17.8	18.4

Calorie Expenditure per Minute for Various Activities

	Body Weight																					
	90	99	108	117	125	134	143	152	161	170	178	187	196	205	213	222	231	240	249	257	266	275
Rowing (recreation)	3.0	3.3	3.6	3.9	4.2	4.5	4.8	5.1	5.4	5.6	6.0	6.2	6.5	6.8	7.1	7.5	7.7	8.0	8.3	8.6	8.9	9.2
Rowing (machine)	8.2	9.0	9.8	10.6	11.4	12.2	13.0	13.8	14.6	15.4	16.2	17.0	17.8	18.6	19.4	20.2	21.0	21.8	22.6	23.4	24.2	25.0
Running, 11-min. mile 5.5 mph	6.4	7.1	7.7	8.3	9.0	9.6	10.2	10.8	11.5	12.1	12.7	13.4	14.0	14.6	15.2	15.9	16.5	17.1	17.8	18.4	19.0	19.6
Running, 8.5-min. mile 7 mph	8.4	9.2	10.0	10.8	11.7	12.5	13.3	14.1	14.9	15.7	16.6	17.4	18.2	19.0	19.8	20.7	21.5	22.3	23.1	23.9	24.8	25.6
Running, 7-min. mile 9 mph	9.3	10.2	11.1	12.9	13.1	13.9	14.8	15.7	16.6	17.5	18.9	19.3	20.2	21.1	22.1	23.0	23.9	24.8	25.7	26.6	27.5	28.4
Running, 5-min. mile 12 mph	11.8	13.0	14.1	15.3	16.4	17.6	18.7	19.9	21.0	22.2	23.3	24.5	25.6	26.8	27.9	29.1	30.2	31.4	32.5	33.7	34.9	36.0
Sailing	1.8	2.0	2.1	2.3	2.4	2.7	2.8	3.0	3.2	3.4	3.6	3.8	3.9	4.1	4.3	4.4	4.6	4.8	5.0	5.1	5.3	5.5
Sit ups	4.3	4.7	5.1	5.6	6.0	6.4	6.8	7.2	7.7	8.1	8.5	8.9	9.4	9.8	10.2	10.6	11.0	11.5	11.9	12.3	12.7	13.2
Sprinting	13.8	15.2	16.6	17.9	19.2	20.5	21.9	23.3	24.7	26.1	27.3	28.7	30.0	31.4	32.7	34.0	35.4	36.8	39.2	39.4	40.3	42.2
Skating (moderate)	3.4	3.8	4.1	4.4	4.8	5.1	5.4	5.8	6.1	6.4	6.8	7.1	7.4	7.8	8.1	8.3	8.8	9.1	9.4	9.8	10.1	10.4
Skating (vigorous)	6.2	6.8	7.4	8.0	8.6	9.2	9.8	9.9	11.0	11.6	12.2	12.8	13.4	14.0	14.6	15.2	15.8	16.4	17.0	17.6	18.2	18.8
Skiing (downhill)	5.8	6.4	6.9	7.5	8.1	8.6	9.2	9.8	10.3	10.9	11.4	12.0	12.6	13.1	13.7	14.3	14.8	15.4	16.0	16.5	17.1	17.7
Skiing (level, 5 mph)	7.0	7.7	8.4	9.1	9.8	10.5	11.1	11.8	12.5	13.2	13.9	14.6	15.2	15.9	16.6	17.3	18.0	18.7	19.4	20.0	20.7	21.4
Skiing (racing downhill)	9.9	10.9	11.9	12.9	13.7	14.7	15.7	16.7	17.7	18.7	19.6	20.6	21.6	22.6	23.4	24.4	25.4	26.4	27.4	28.3	29.3	30.2
Snowshoeing (2.3 mph)	3.7	4.1	4.5	4.8	5.2	5.5	5.9	6.3	6.7	7.0	7.4	7.8	8.1	8.5	8.8	9.2	9.6	9.9	10.3	10.6	11.0	11.4
Snowshoeing (2.5 mph)	5.4	5.9	6.5	7.0	7.5	8.0	8.6	9.1	9.7	10.2	10.7	11.2	11.6	12.1	12.7	13.2	13.9	14.3	14.9	15.4	16.0	16.5
Soccer	5.4	5.9	6.4	6.9	7.5	8.0	8.5	9.0	9.6	10.1	10.6	11.1	11.6	12.1	12.7	13.2	13.4	14.3	14.8	15.3	15.8	16.9
Squash	6.2	6.8	7.5	8.1	8.7	9.3	9.9	10.5	11.1	11.7	12.3	12.9	13.5	14.2	14.8	15.4	16.0	16.7	17.2	17.8	18.4	19.0
Stationary Running, 140 counts/min.	14.6	16.1	17.5	18.9	20.4	21.8	23.2	24.6	26.1	27.5	28.9	30.4	31.8	33.2	34.6	36.1	37.5	38.9	40.4	41.8	43.2	44.6
Swimming, pleasure 25 yds./min.	3.6	4.0	4.3	4.7	5.0	5.4	5.7	6.1	6.4	6.8	7.1	7.5	7.8	8.2	8.5	8.9	9.2	9.6	10.0	10.3	10.6	11.0
Swimming, back 20 yds./min.	2.3	2.6	2.8	3.0	3.2	3.5	3.7	3.9	4.1	4.2	4.6	4.8	5.0	5.3	5.5	5.7	6.0	6.2	6.4	6.6	6.9	7.1
Swimming, back 30 yds./min.	3.2	3.5	3.8	4.1	4.4	4.7	5.1	5.4	5.7	6.0	6.3	6.6	6.9	7.2	7.4	7.9	8.2	8.5	8.8	9.1	9.4	9.7
Swimming, back 40 yds./min.	5.0	5.5	5.8	6.5	7.0	7.5	7.9	8.5	8.9	9.4	9.9	10.4	10.9	11.4	11.9	12.3	12.8	13.3	13.8	14.3	14.8	15.3
Swimming, breast 20 yds./min.	2.9	3.2	3.4	3.8	4.0	4.3	4.6	4.9	5.1	5.4	5.7	6.0	6.3	6.5	6.8	7.1	7.4	7.7	7.9	8.2	8.5	8.8
Swimming, breast 30 yds./min.	4.3	4.8	5.2	5.7	6.0	6.4	6.9	7.3	7.7	8.1	8.6	9.0	9.4	9.9	10.3	10.8	11.1	11.5	11.9	12.4	13.0	13.3
Swimming, breast 40 yds./min.	5.8	6.3	6.9	7.5	8.0	8.6	9.2	9.7	10.3	10.8	11.4	12.0	12.5	13.1	13.7	14.2	14.8	15.4	15.9	16.5	17.0	17.6

Calorie Expenditure per Minute for Various Activities

	Body Weight																					
	90	99	108	117	125	134	143	152	161	170	178	187	196	205	213	222	231	240	249	257	266	275
Swimming, butterfly 50 yds./min.	7.0	7.7	8.4	9.1	9.8	10.5	11.1	11.9	12.5	13.2	13.9	14.6	15.2	15.9	16.6	17.3	18.0	18.7	19.4	20.0	20.7	21.4
Swimming, crawl 20 yds./min.	2.9	3.2	3.4	3.8	4.0	4.3	4.6	4.9	5.1	5.4	5.7	5.8	6.3	6.5	6.8	7.1	7.3	7.7	7.9	8.2	8.5	8.8
Swimming, crawl 45 yds./min.	5.2	5.8	6.3	6.8	7.3	7.8	8.3	8.8	9.3	9.8	10.4	10.9	11.4	11.9	12.4	12.9	13.4	13.9	14.4	15.0	15.5	16.0
Swimming, crawl 50 yds./min.	6.4	7.0	7.6	8.3	8.9	9.5	10.1	10.7	11.4	12.0	12.6	13.2	13.9	14.5	15.1	15.7	16.3	17.0	17.4	17.9	18.8	19.5
Table Tennis	2.3	2.6	2.8	3.0	3.2	3.5	3.7	3.9	4.1	4.2	4.6	4.8	5.0	5.3	5.5	5.7	6.0	6.2	6.4	6.6	6.9	7.1
Tennis (recreation)	4.2	4.6	5.0	5.4	5.8	6.2	6.6	7.0	7.4	7.8	8.2	8.6	9.0	9.4	9.8	10.2	10.6	11.0	11.5	11.9	12.3	12.6
Tennis (competition)	5.9	6.4	7.0	7.6	8.1	8.7	9.3	9.9	10.4	11.0	11.6	12.1	12.7	13.3	13.9	14.4	15.0	15.6	16.1	16.7	17.3	17.9
Timed Calisthenics	8.8	9.6	10.5	11.4	12.2	13.1	13.9	14.8	15.6	16.5	17.4	18.2	19.1	19.9	20.8	21.5	22.5	23.4	24.2	25.1	25.9	26.8
Volleyball (moderate)	3.4	3.8	4.0	4.4	4.8	5.1	5.4	5.8	6.1	6.4	6.8	7.1	7.4	7.8	8.1	8.3	8.8	9.1	9.4	9.8	10.1	10.4
Volleyball (vigorous)	5.9	6.4	7.0	7.6	8.1	8.7	9.3	9.9	10.4	11.0	11.6	12.1	12.7	13.3	13.9	14.4	15.0	15.6	16.1	16.7	17.3	17.9
Walking (2.0 mph)	2.1	2.3	2.5	2.7	2.9	3.1	3.3	3.5	3.7	4.0	4.2	4.4	4.6	4.8	5.0	5.2	5.4	5.6	5.8	6.0	6.2	6.4
Walking (4.5 mph)	4.0	4.4	4.7	5.1	5.5	5.9	6.3	6.7	7.1	7.5	7.8	8.2	8.6	9.0	9.4	9.8	10.1	10.6	10.9	11.3	11.7	12.0
Walking 110-120 steps/min.	3.1	3.4	3.7	4.0	4.3	4.7	5.0	5.3	5.6	5.9	6.2	6.5	6.8	7.1	7.4	7.7	8.0	8.3	8.6	8.9	9.2	9.5
Waterskiing	4.7	5.1	5.6	6.1	6.5	7.0	7.4	7.9	8.3	8.8	9.3	9.7	10.2	10.6	11.1	11.5	12.0	12.5	12.9	13.4	13.8	14.3
Weight Training	4.7	5.1	5.7	6.2	6.7	7.0	7.5	7.9	8.4	8.9	9.4	9.9	10.3	10.8	11.1	11.7	12.2	12.6	13.1	13.5	14.0	14.4
Wrestling	7.7	8.5	9.2	10.0	10.7	11.5	12.2	13.0	13.7	14.5	15.2	16.0	16.7	17.5	18.2	19.0	19.7	20.5	21.2	22.0	22.7	23.5

From Consolazio, Johnson and Pecora, Physiological Measurements of Metabolic Functions in Man, McGraw-Hill, 1963.

GOING BEYOND
■
Lab Reports

LAB 1

STUDENT CONSENT FORM

As a student in this exercise course you will be involved in several exercise conditioning and testing programs.

A series of tests has been designed to determine the status of various personal health factors. All results will be used as base data to establish training programs related to modification and improvement of each individual's fitness, muscle tone and body proportions.

The activities which will be used to reach the student's objectives as determined by pre-tests, include:

1. jog and walk
2. jump rope activity
3. isometrics
4. weight training
5. correctives for posture
6. progressive relaxation
7. circuit training
8. aqua dynamics
9. aerobic dance
10. RCAF Fitness program
11. additional selections

In signing this consent form you state that you have read and understand the nature of these activities. You furthermore state that you are entering into these activities of your own free will and that you may withdraw from participation at any time. Assuredly, every effort will be made to insure your safe participation in this class. All activity will be performed within your personal limitations and capabilities.

Please indicate any medical related problems or other conditions that need to be considered in developing a personal health program for you.

Name of Family Physician _____

Name of Applicant (print) _____

Signature of Applicant _____

Address _____

Phone _____

Student Number _____

Indicate medical limitations _____

_____

_____

LAB 2
PRE-EXERCISE MEDICAL HISTORY FORM

NAME _____ AGE _____ DATE _____

ADDRESS _____ PHONE _____

OCCUPATION _____ HT _____ WT _____

DOCTOR'S NAME _____ PHONE _____

Past History (Mark X if Yes)

(Have you ever had?)   **Dates**

Diabetes ( ) _____
Rheumatic Fever ( ) _____
Heart Murmur ( ) _____
High Blood Pressure ( ) _____
Any Heart Trouble ( ) _____
Disease of Arteries ( ) _____
Varicose Veins ( ) _____
Lung Disease ( ) _____
Operations ( ) _____
Epilepsy ( ) _____
Cancer ( ) _____
Anemia ( ) _____
Injuries to Back, Knees, ( ) _____
  Ankles, etc.
Explain:

Family History (Have any of your relatives had?)

                                      Age   **Relative**

Heart Attacks ( ) _____ _____
High Blood Pressure ( ) _____ _____
High Cholesterol Levels ( ) _____ _____
Diabetes ( ) _____ _____
Congenital Heart Diseases ( ) _____ _____
Heart Operations ( ) _____ _____
Cancer ( ) _____ _____
Stroke ( ) _____ _____
Other: ( ) _____ _____

Explain:

Present Symptoms Review

(Have you recently had?)   **Date**

Chest Pain ( ) _____
Shortness of Breath ( ) _____
Heart Palpitations ( ) _____
Cough on Exertion ( ) _____

Explain:

                                      Date
Coughing of Blood ( ) _____
Back Pain ( ) _____
Swollen, Stiff or Painful Joints ( ) _____

Risk Factors

1. **Smoking**   Yes No

   Cigarettes ( ) ( )   How many?_____ How many years?_____

   Cigar   ( ) ( )   How many?_____ How many years? _____

   Pipe   ( ) ( )   How many times a day?_____ How many years?_____

   How old were you when you started?_____

   In case you have stopped, when did you?_____

   Why?_____ _____

2. **Diet**

   What is your weight now?_____ 1 year ago?_____ At age 21?_____

   Are you dieting?_____ Why?_____

3. **Exercise**

   Do you engage in any exercise, fitness, or recreational activities?_____

   What?_____ How often?_____

   How far do you think you walk each day?_____

   Is your occupation:

Sedentary	( )	Active	( )
Inactive	( )	Heavy Work	( )

   Do you have discomfort, shortness of breath, or pain with moderate exercise?_____

   Were you a high school or college athlete?_____ Specify_____

Mark any of the medicines you are now taking

   _____ Mood elevators (pills for depression)

   _____ Pep or diet pills (like dexadrine)

   _____ Tranquilizers, sedatives, nerve or sleeping pills (Miltown, Librium, Phenobarbital, Nembutal, Seconal, etc.)

   _____ Pain pills (Demerol, Codeine, Morphine, etc.)

   _____ Antihistamines or allergy pills

   _____ Blood pressure pills

LAB 3
FITNESS PROFILE CHART

NAME_____ SECTION_____DATE _____

FITNESS TEST	Initial Score	Rating	Final Score	Rating	Change
CARDIOVASCULAR					
Resting Heart Rate					
Walking Test					
Sit/Stand Test					
12 Min. Run/1.5 Mile Run					
FLEXIBILITY					
Bend and Reach					
Shoulder Lift					
Trunk Extension					
MUSCULAR ENDURANCE					
Sit-Ups					
Push-Ups					
Static Push-Up					

198

Conclusions:

Initial Tests

What do the initial tests indicate as your area of greatest weakness?

Area of greatest strength?

Final Tests

1. In which areas did you show significant improvement?

2. What were the reasons for your areas of improvement?

3. If you did not improve on any of the tests what do you think is the reason?

4. What implications do your results have for the future?

LAB 4
CONTRACT FOR CHANGE

NAME _____SECTION _____DATE _____

Establishing goals for change is an important process. Individuals must determine the changes they desire and make a plan as to how best achieve these changes. By your commitment this endeavor could bring about lifestyle changes.

Procedure:

Indicate the goals that you currently desire to achieve during the next semester. Be specific within each general area.

| **Goal** | **Steps to Reach the Goal** |

1. **Fitness**

    A.   Cardiovascular Endurance

    B.   Flexibility

    C.   Muscular Endurance

2. **Body Composition**

    A.   Weight

    B.   Body Fat Percentage

3. **Body Measurements**

4. **Posture**

Conclusions

1. Which goals do you feel will be the most difficult for you to achieve?

2. What type of assistance do you need to help you achieve these goals?

3. Do you feel you are well motivated to achieve these goals?

LAB 5
ANALYSIS OF BODY FAT PERCENTAGES

NAME _____ SECTION _____ DATE _____

Determination of the percentage of body fat can be made by measurement with a skinfold caliper. A pinch of skin is pulled away from the underlying muscle and the thickness of the fold is measured with the caliper.

Results: Skinfold Measurements

FEMALES

Triceps (arm) _____

Abdomen _____

Hip (Ilium) _____

TOTAL _____

MALES

Chest _____

Hip (Ilium) _____

Abdomen _____

Side (Axilla) _____

TOTAL _____

Percentage of Body Fat: (See Appendix A)

Sum of all Scores = _____

Rating of Individual Measurements

FEMALES

Triceps _____

Abdomen _____

Hip (Ilium) _____

TOTAL _____

MALES

Chest _____

Hip (Ilium) _____

Abdomen _____

Side (Axilla) _____

TOTAL _____

Average of Scores = _____

Rating   = _____

Conclusions:

1. How does your percentage of body fat compare with the optimal percentage (15 % for males, 20 % for females)?

2. What implications do these results have for improvement of your body composition?

LAB 6
ANALYSIS OF BODY COMPOSITION

NAME_____ SECTION_____ DATE_____

Age_____Height _____Target Weight _____

Initial **Body Weight** _____Final Body Weight_____Change_____

Initial **Body Fat %**_____Final Body Fat %_____Change_____

GIRTH MEASUREMENTS

Site	Initial Score	Desirable Score	Final Score	Actual Change
Chest (Bust)				
Waist				
Abdomen				
Hips				
Thigh: right				
left				
Calf: right				
left				
Ankle: right				
left				
Upper arm: right				
left				
Wrist				

Conclusions:

Initial Tests

What do the initial tests indicate as your areas of greatest concern?

Final Tests

1. In which areas did you show significant improvement?

2. Which areas do you feel still need improvement?

3. What implications do your results have for the future?

LAB 7
NUTRITION AND DIET ANALYSIS

NAME_____ SECTION_____ DATE_____

Procedure:

1. Record everything you eat or drink for ten days on the chart provided. Record what was consumed, how much, and the time of day. Eat as normally as you can.

2. Using Appendix F, estimate the number of calories, grams of carbohydrates, protein, and fat, and intake of the designated vitamins and minerals.

Analysis:

1. Total all columns for each day and for the ten-day period.

2. Total all calories for each meal for each day.

3. Transfer figures to Diet Recall Summary Form.

4. Determine the average daily intake in all columns by dividing by 10.

5. Determine average calories from fat, protein, and carbohydrate by multiplying the daily average by 9, 4, & 4 respectively.

6. Determine percent of carbohydrate, fat, and protein intake by dividing total calories into daily average in area and compare with optimal.

7. Compare your intake of vitamins and minerals with the RDA.

Conclusions

1. On how many days out of the ten did you eat properly from the four basic food groups?

2. Which group do you tend to omit?

3. In which group do you tend to overeat?

4. How did your percentage of proteins, carbohydrates and fats compare with the optimal amount recommended?

5. What was the highest calorie food per serving that you ate or drank?

6. Which food gave you the highest amount of saturated fat?

7. When do you tend to eat the most calories?

8. What empty calories (no nutritional value) did you consume?

9. Do you snack? How much? What?

10. Could you include more healthful snacks? What?

11. Do you drink enough fluids daily?

12. On the basis of this analysis, what specific recommendations do you have regarding your current eating habits (foods you need to eliminate or cut back on, foods you need to eat more, low-calorie snacks you could select, etc.)

LABORATORY 7, *CONTINUED*

NAME_____SECTION_____ DATE_____

Day	Time	Food	Amount	Calories	Protein Grams	Fat	Saturated Fat	Unsaturated Fat	Carbohydrates	Calcium	Phosphorus	Iron	Potassium	Vitamin A	Thiamin	Riboflavin	Niacin	Vitamin C

Day	Time	Food	Amount	Calories	Protein Grams	Fat	Saturated Fat	Unsaturated Fat	Carbohydrates	Calcium	Phosphorus	Iron	Potassium	Vitamin A	Thiamin	Riboflavin	Niacin	Vitamin C

LABORATORY 7, *CONTINUED*

NAME_____SECTION_____ DATE_____

1. Calorie Analysis (Totals for each meal)

Days	1	2	3	4	5	6	7	8	9	10
Breakfast										
Lunch										
Dinner										
Snacks										
TOTALS										

2. Total Nutrients for 10 Days

A. Total calories_____

B. Total grams of protein_____

C. Total grams of fat_____

D. Total grams of saturated fat_____

E. Total grams of unsaturated fat_____

F. Total grams of carbohydrates_____

3. Average Nutrients per Day (Divide above by 10)

A. Average calories_____

B. Average grams of protein_____

C. Average grams of fat_____

D. Average grams of saturated fat_____

E. Average grams of unsaturated fat_____

F. Average grams of carbohydrates_____

4. **Average Calories Per Day Per Nutrient**

   A. Multiply average grams of protein per day by 4

   B. Multiply average grams of fat by 9

   C. Multiply average grams of saturated fat by 9

   D. Multiply average grams of unsaturated fat by 9

   E. Multiply average grams of carbohydrates by 4

5. **Percentage of Calories from Each Nutrient**

   A. Divide average calories per day from protein by average total calories per day.

   Total calories per day _____) Calories from protein

   B. Divide average calories per day from fat by average total calories per day.

   Total calories per day _____) Calories from fat

   C. Divide average calories per day from unsaturated fat by average total calories per day.

   Total calories per day _____) Calories from unsaturated fat

   D. Divide average calories per day from saturated fat by average total calories per day.

   Total calories per day _____) Calories from saturated fat

   E. Divide average calories per day from carbohydrates by average total calories per day.

   Total calories per day _____) Calories from carbohydrates

LAB 8
WEIGHT CONTROL CONTRACT

NAME_____ SECTION_____ DATE_____

Calorie Expenditure

1. Exercise Preference_____

2. Calories extended per minute (see Appendix J)_____

3. Number of minutes to exercise each day_____

4. Calories expended per day (line 2 × line 3)_____

Calorie Intake

5. Average caloric intake (from Lab 7 — Nutrition and Diet)_____

6. Calorie reduction per day to lose 2 pounds per week

   − 1,000 _____

7. Total daily calorie intake, without exercise 2 pounds a week

   (line 5 − line 6) _____

8. Daily calorie intake to lose 2 pounds per week, including exercise

   (line 7 + line 4)_____

   (*Note:* This total should not be below 1200 calories for women or 1500 calories for men.)

Contract Agreement

Height _____ Present weight _____ Target weight _____

My goal is to lose (gain) _____ pounds in _____ weeks. _____

_____   _____   _____
Signature   Date   Approval

_____   _____   _____
Contract Completion Date   Weight   Actual Change

WEEKLY WEIGHT RECORD

Weeks

	1	2	3	4	5	6	7	8	9	10	11	12	13	14	15	16
1																
2																
3																
4																
5																
6																
7																
8																
9																
10																
11																
12																
13																
14																
15																
16																
17																
18																
19																
20																

Weight change in pounds

LAB 9
TARGET HEART RATE ZONE

NAME_____ SECTION_____DATE_____

Target heart rate zone identifies for each person the safe and comfortable area in which cardiovascular exercise should occur to achieve a training effect.

Procedure

1. First, you must determine your maximum heart rate according to your age.

   The formula is: 220 – Age = Maximum Heart Rate.

   Example: 220
   $$\frac{-19}{201}\ \text{MHR}$$

   It is not safe for you to work at a rate this high. Therefore, we must identify your TARGET HEART RATE ZONE, the safe upper limit and minimum lower limit necessary for cardiovascular improvement to occur.

2 . It is important to consider your current resting heart rate because that is your individual starting point during exercise.

   201 (MHR) – Resting Heart Rate = Heart Rate Reserve
   Example: 201 (MHR)
   $$\frac{-68\ \text{(RHR)}}{133}\ \text{Heart Rate Reserve}$$

3. The lower limit for a training effect is 70%:

   133 (Heart Rate Reserve) × .70 + RHR = Target Zone Lower Limit
   Example: 133
   .70
   93.10
   $$\frac{+68}{161.10}\ \text{RHR}$$
   = Target Zone Lower Limit

4. The safe upper limit is 85%:

   133 (Heart Rate Reserve) × .85 + RHR = Target Zone Upper Limit
   Example: 133
   .85
   113.05
   $$\frac{+68.00}{181.05}\ \text{RHR}$$
   Target Zone Upper Limit

Assignment: Using the formula described above, compute your target heart rate for the 70% and 85% limits, using the form provided on the next page.

Lower Limit	Upper Limit
220	220
_____	_____
_____	_____
_____	_____
_____	_____
.70	.85
_____	_____
_____	_____
_____	_____

Conclusions:

1. What is your 10 second pulse count for your lower limit?_____
   For your upper limit?_____

2. What should you do if you find that you are not reaching your lower limit?

3. What should you do if you find that you are exceeding your upper limit?

LAB 10
EXERCISE RECORDING FORM

NAME_____ SECTION_____ DATE_____

Target Heart Rate: Lower Limit_____Upper Limit _____

| DATE | FITNESS AREA | TYPE OF EXERCISE | ACTUAL WORKOUT TIME | HEART RATE | | | CALORIES BURNED |
				PRE EX.	POST EX.	FIVE MIN.	

LAB 11
BLOOD PRESSURE RECORD

NAME_____ SECTION_____ DATE_____

Blood pressure is a record of the pressure generated by the outflow of blood against the arterial walls. The highest reading is the **systolic** and represents peak pressure in your arteries during the contraction phase of the heart. The lowest pressure in the arteries is the **diastolic** and represents the pressure during the relaxation phase. The acceptable range for your blood pressure is stated as

SYSTOLIC = 120 ± 20 or 100 – 140

DIASTOLIC = 80 ± 10 or 70 – 90

Assignment:

Secure a record of your blood pressure for five days from any reliable source: doctor, nurse, school nurse, athletic trainer, home blood pressure unit, school fitness lab, etc.

Results:

	DATE	TIME	BLOOD PRESSURE READING	WHERE CHECKED
1.				
2.				
3.				
4.				
5.				

Conclusions:

1. What is your typical blood pressure?

2. Does your blood pressure level indicate you are at a safe level?

3. What might cause fluctuations or variations in one's blood pressure?

Lab 12 RISKO — Heart Attack Risk Factors

NAME_____ SECTION_____ DATE_____

The purpose of this game is to give you an estimate of your chances of suffering heart attack. The game is played by marking squares which — from left to right — represent an increase in your *risk factors*. These are medical conditions and habits associated with an increased danger of heart attack. Not all risk factors are measurable enough to be included in this game.

Rules:

Study each risk factor and its row. Find the box applicable to you and circle the large number in it. For example, if you are 37, circle the number in the box labeled 31-40.

After checking out all the rows, add the circled numbers. This total — your score — is an estimate of your risk.

If You Score:

6-11 — Risk well below average

12-17 — Risk below average

18-24 — Risk generally average

25-31 — Risk moderate

32-40 — Risk at a dangerous level

41-62 — Danger urgent. See your doctor now.

Heredity:

Count parents, grandparents, brothers, and sisters who have had heart attack and/or stroke.

Tobacco Smoking:

If you inhale deeply and smoke a cigarette way down, add one to your classification. Do *not* subtract because you think you do not inhale or smoke only a half inch on a cigarette.

Exercise:

Lower your score one point if you exercise regularly and frequently.

Cholesterol or Saturated Fat Intake Level:

A cholesterol blood level is best. If you can't get one from your doctor, then estimate honestly the percentage of solid fats you eat. These are usually of animal origin — lard, cream, butter, and beef and lamb fat. If you eat much of this, your cholesterol level probably will be high. The United States average, 40 percent, is too high for good health.

Blood Pressure:

If you have no recent reading but have passed an insurance or industrial examination chances are you are 140 or less.

Sex:

This line takes into account the fact that men have from 6 to 10 times more heart attacks than women of child bearing age.

AGE	10 to 20	21 to 30	31 to 40	41 to 50	51 to 60	61 to 70
HEREDITY	No known history of heart disease	1 relative with cardiovascular disease Over 60	2 relatives with cardiovascular disease Over 60	1 relative with cardiovascular disease Under 60	2 relatives with cardiovascular disease Under 60	3 relatives with cardiovascular disease Under 60
WEIGHT	More than 5 lbs. below standard weight	−5 to + 5 lbs standard weight	6-20 lbs over weight	21-35 lbs over weight	36-50 lbs over weight	51-65 lbs over weight
TOBACCO SMOKING	Non-user	Cigar and/or pipe	10 cigarettes or less a day	20 cigarettes a day	30 cigarettes a day	40 cigarettes a day or more
EXERCISE	Intensive occupational and recreational exertion	Moderate occupational and recreational exertion	Sedentary work and intense recreational exertion	Sedentary occupational and moderate exertion	Sedentary work and light recreational	Complete lack of all exercise
CHOLES-TEROL OR FAT % IN DIET	Cholesterol below 180 mg % Diet contains no animal or solid fats	Cholesterol 181-205 mg % Diet contains 10% animal or solid fats	Cholesterol 206-230 mg % Diet contains 20% animal or solid fats	Cholesterol 231-255 mg % Diet contains 30% animal or solid fats	Cholesterol 256-280 mg % Diet contains 40% animal or solid fats	Cholesterol 281-300 mg % Diet contains 50% animal or solid fats
BLOOD PRESSURE	100 upper reading	120 upper reading	140 upper reading	160 upper reading	180 upper reading	200 or over upper reading
SEX	Female under 40	Female 40-50	Female over 50	Male	Stocky male	Bald stocky male

For meaningful interpretation of RISKO only the official RISKO directions should be used.

Conclusions:

1. What is your total score?

2. What is your classification?

3. What does this indicate you should do to lower your heart attack risk?

LAB 13
POSTURE ANALYSIS

NAME _____ SECTION _____ DATE _____

Posture refers to the position assumed by the body. Good posture is important for appearance, for maximal movement efficiency, to prevent soreness and muscle strains, and to enhance function of internal organs. If deviations from proper alignment are noted, it may be possible to suggest exercises to correct the problem.

Procedure

1. Have a partner assist you by comparing your alignment of various body areas with those on the Posture Rating Chart.

2. Record the score which best corresponds to your rating.

Posture Rating Chart (see next page)

Conclusions:

1. Is there a particular area of your body that seems to need improved alignment?

2. What specific exercises would be appropriate to improve your posture?

3. Do you feel you need qualified professional help to assist you?

POSTURE SCORE SHEET				SCORING DATES		
Name _____						
	GOOD – 10	**FAIR – 5**	**POOR – 0**			
HEAD LEFT RIGHT	HEAD ERECT GRAVITY LINE PASSES DIRECTLY THROUGH CENTER	HEAD TWISTED OR TURNED TO ONE SIDE SLIGHTLY	HEAD TWISTED OR TURNED TO ONE SIDE MARKEDLY			
SHOULDERS LEFT RIGHT	SHOULDERS LEVEL (HORIZONTALLY)	ONE SHOULDER SLIGHTLY HIGHER THAN OTHER	ONE SHOULDER MARKEDLY HIGHER THAN OTHER			
SPINE LEFT RIGHT	SPINE STRAIGHT	SPINE SLIGHTLY CURVED LATERALLY	SPINE MARKEDLY CURVED LATERALLY			
HIPS LEFT RIGHT	HIPS LEVEL (HORIZONTALLY)	ONE HIP SLIGHTLY HIGHER	ONE HIP MARKEDLY HIGHER			
ANKLES	FEET POINTED STRAIGHT AHEAD	FEET POINTED OUT	FEET POINTED OUT MARKEDLY ANKLES SAG IN (PRONATION)			
NECK	NECK ERECT, CHIN IN, HEAD IN BALANCE DIRECTLY ABOVE SHOULDERS	NECK SLIGHTLY FORWARD CHIN SLIGHTLY OUT	NECK MARKEDLY FORWARD, CHIN MARKEDLY OUT			
UPPER BACK	UPPER BACK NORMALLY ROUNDED	UPPER BACK SLIGHTLY MORE ROUNDED	UPPER BACK MARKEDLY ROUNDED			
TRUNK	TRUNK ERECT	TRUNK INCLINED TO REAR SLIGHTLY	TRUNK INCLINED TO REAR MARKEDLY			
ABDOMEN	ABDOMEN FLAT	ABDOMEN PROTRUDING	ABDOMEN PROTRUDING AND SAGGING			
LOWER BACK	LOWER BACK NORMALLY CURVED	LOWER BACK SLIGHTLY HOLLOW	LOWER BACK MARKEDLY HOLLOW			
			TOTAL SCORES			

Source: Reedco, Inc., Auburn, NY

LAB 14
STRESS ASSESSMENT

NAME_____SECTION_____DATE _____

Purpose:

1. To assist you in evaluating your degree of stress and tension.

2. To alert you to certain stress symptoms in your life which indicate a need for stress reduction techniques.

Procedure:

Answer the following questions and score yourself.

A Checklist to Determine Tenseness

YES	NO	At TIMES	
( )	( )	( )	1. Do you frequently have trouble falling asleep?
( )	( )	( )	2. Do you frequently experience headaches or backaches?
( )	( )	( )	3. Do you frequently feel "uptight" at the end of the day?
( )	( )	( )	4. Do you frequently lose your patience when others are late?
( )	( )	( )	5. Do you frequently complain of being tired?
( )	( )	( )	6. Are you unable to shut out your worries when you go to bed at night?
( )	( )	( )	7. Are you unable to release tensions even when you are aware of them?
( )	( )	( )	8. Are you frequently concerned by time pressures and deadlines?
( )	( )	( )	9. Are you highly competitive in most areas of your life: sports, test grades, and daily responsibilities?
( )	( )	( )	10. Are you too busy to plan time for exercise or physical activity?
( )	( )	( )	11. Are you upset when your plans are interrupted or must be changed?

Scoring: After checking each question give yourself a + 1 for every NO answer; a − 1 for every YES answer; and a − ½ for every At Times answer.

+	−
8-11 *"Far Out Man or Lady"*	8-11 *"Like a Clock Spring"*
5-7 *Loose*	5-7 *Tense*
3-4 *Above Average Looseness*	3-4 *Above Average Tenseness*
1-2 *Average Looseness*	1-2 *Average Tenseness*

Results:

1. What is your total score?_____

2. What is your stress level according to the test?_____

Conclusions and Implications:

1. What changes in your lifestyle might help lower your stress?

2. What techniques might be used to help you learn to relax?

LAB 15
AEROBIC DANCE WORKOUT

NAME_____ SECTION_____ DATE_____

Purpose

1. To give you an opportunity to acquire a learning experience in aerobic dance fitness.

2. To provide you with a sequential routine of dance steps and patterns that have been selected to work you out in a cardiovascular style.

3. To acquaint you with a dance exercise program that you might wish to maintain throughout your life.

Procedure

Warm up sufficiently in order to perform the following dance steps and patterns. It is suggested that this designed sequence be followed in the exact progression as listed.

You will notice that the format begins gradually, becomes progressively more difficult, has interludes of stretching, reaches a high workout peak, and then diminishes to a slower, more controlled pace once again.

The following aerobic dance progression is paced for a beginning level workout. You may expend your energy level through one of the following workout channels:

Low channel: Minimal walking or shuffling.
Medium channel: Soft bouncy jogging.
High channel: High jogging and exaggerated range of body movements.

You might even wish to consider employing a flow of exchange between one energy level and another; pace yourself for a good workout! Also, it is important to note that you must be well into a condition of fitness which adequately allows you to assume a target heart rate score.

Furthermore, be sure to plan your cool-down activity to include sufficient walking and stretching time.

Prepare yourself by reading Chapter 5 on Aerobic Dance. Acquaint yourself with the terminology and execution of the dance steps and patterns in Chapter 5 and the warm-up and cool-down in Chapter 6. Background music may be played in the classroom and/or at home for rhythmic enjoyment. Select a dance partner and have this person call out verbal commands to you as he or she reads from the step format. Your partner should give you ongoing cues so as not to delay or interrupt your total workout time schedule. Upon completing your lab assignment, you should then exchange partnership role responsibility.

The Warm-up (Approx. 10 minutes)

(A) Allow 3 minutes light workout.

(B) Allow 3 minutes stretching.

(C) Allow 1 minute light workout.

Note: Check heart rate immediately after finishing the warm-up.

The Workout (Approx. 7 minutes)

(D) Eccentric steps R 8 — — — — — — — — —
Grapevine L clap, grapevine R clap
Jump - clap side to side 16
Repeat 2nd time   2x
Repeat 3rd time
Slides R 8, L 8, R 8, L 8 — — — — — — — —

(E) Scissors — doubles fwd-bkwd 4 — — — — — —
Scissors — singles fwd-bkwd 8
Jog square to R 8
Jog square to R 8
Jog square to R 8   2x
Jog square to R 8
Break — 2 slow, 3 quicks
Break — 2 slow, 3 quicks — — — — — — — —

(F) R Polka heel-toe 2 x slide R 4 — — — — — — — — — —
L Polka heel-toe 2 x slide L 4
R Polka heel-toe 2 x slide R 4
L Polka heel-toe 2 x slide L 4
Double drop arm swings 4, R, L, R, L   2x
Body waist drop swing R, archery bow pull L lean back
Double drop arm swing 4 R, L, R, L
Body waist drop swing L, archery bow pull R lean back — — —

(G) Hop scotch 4 — — — — — — — — — — — —
Rocks and punches side to side 8
Hops with knee cross overs 8 R
Rocks and punches side to side 8
Hop scotch 4   2x
Rocks and punches side to side 8
Hops with knee cross overs 8 L
Rocks and punches — — — — — — — — — —

(H) Lunge forward — pull back — — — — — — — — — — — — — ⌐
Snap jump, hop knee lift R, snap jump hop knee lift L, 8 x
Can can knee prances 8
Jog heel slaps 8   2x
Break — 2 s, 3 q
Break — 2 s, 3 q — — — — — — — — — — — — — — — — ⌐

(I) Slides R 4, jump fwd, jump bkwd, jump fwd, jump bkwd — — — — ⌐
Slides L 4, jump fwd, jump bkwd, jump fwd, jump bkwd
Slides R 4, jump fwd, jump bkwd, jump fwd, jump bkwd
Slides L 4, jump fwd, jump bkwd, jump fwd, jump bkwd
Pony two steps side to side 4 x   2x
Jog a figure 8 "Hey"
Pony two steps side to side 4 x
Jog a figure 8 "Hey" — — — — — — — — — — — — — — — ⌐

(J) Squat walks 8 forward, grapevine R clap, grapevine L clap — — — ⌐
Repeat 3 x more walking in a square   2x
One arm windups 8 R, 8 L, 8 R, 8 L — — — — — — — — — — ⌐

The Interval Stretching Time (Approx. 1 minute)

(K) Calf stretch R — — — — — — — ⌐
Ball of foot tug R
Calf stretch L
Ball of foot tug L   2x
Thigh stretch quad R
Thigh stretch quad L — — — — ⌐

Shake out gently

The Dancing Down (Approx. 1 minute)

(L) Knee-squat bounce 4 invert, stretch 4 — — — — — — — — — — — ⌐
Knee-squat bounce 4 invert, stretch 4
R straddle bent knee-elbow touch, "X" stretch up; repeat L
Double knee elbow touch, "X" stretch up; repeat
Repeat combination 2 times more   2x
Knee squat to knee stand quad hurdler's stretch, R
Knee squat to knee stand quad hurdler's stretch, L
Sit down — bent knee position — — — — — — — — — — — — — ⌐

> *Note:* Check heart rate before beginning the floor exercises.

The En bas (Approx. 10 minutes)

(M) Rhythmic sit-ups (touch toes, knees, roll down, roll up-snap)
Opp. elbow-knee touch R, L:
Repeat sequence for rhythmic sit-ups and elbow-knee touch combo 25-50 times

(N) Rolli-polli hip twists 24 — bent line
Front leg raises, 16 R, 16 L
Leg scissors lifts 8 - 24 times

(O) Rolli-polli hip twists 24 - long line
Side leg raises 16 R, 16 L
Leg slicer swing-thrus, 8 - 24 on R and L

(P) "Buns up" — hip table top lifts 4 slow 16 fasts
Repeat "buns up" — hip table top lifts 4 slow 16 fasts
Inner thigh lifts 24 R, L
Tight tuck hold, total stretch

The Interval Stretching Time (Approx. 1 minute)

(Q) Long line knee pulses (raisers)
Long line leg raisers (flex foot)
Long line knee and ankle (flex and extend)
Work each leg carefully
Repeat (K) on bar

(Adapt the interval stretching series for floor work.)

The Dancing Up (Approx. 1 minute)

(R) Knee-squat bounce 4 invert, stretch 4
Knee-squat bounce 4 invert, stretch 4
Inchworm walk-out, hold
Runner's stretch with alternating heel lifting in place 16 — 2x
Inchworm walk back
Spine roll up
Spine roll down
Spine roll up

The Workout (Approx. 1 minute)

(S) Repeat (G)

(T) Repeat (H)

(U) Repeat (I)

(V) Repeat (J)

Interval Stretch (Approx. 1 minute)

(W) Repeat (K)

Tapering (Approx. 1 minute)

(X) March fwd 8
     March bkwd 8
     Squat walk in a circle 16
     Repeat 3 more times
     Stretch ups — side to side stepping in place (oppositional rib and hip action) 16
     Total body alignment stretch up and hold

Note: (Check heart rate immediately after completing this program.)

The Cool-down (Approx. 3 minutes)

(Y) Allow 1 minute stretching à Terre.

(Z_1) Allow 1 minute stretching en bas.

(Z_2) Allow 1 minute stretching en bas at wall.

Results

1. Were you able to perform efficiently all the dance steps and patterns in the workout program? _____ If not, which ones were you unable to perform?

2. Did you stretch out sufficiently enough for your own needs during the time of:

   A. warm up

   B. interludes

   C. cool-down

3. Did you maintain your exercise pulse level during the pulse check intervals?

4. Did you reach your Target Heart Rate during the pulse check readings?

5. What energy level did you utilize? _____ Did you incorporate more than one level? _____ When? _____ How often? _____

Conclusions and Implications

1. Is this a suitable style of cardiovascular work out for you?

2. Did you receive a good work out from this program? Why or why not?

3. What could you do to make the program more difficult? More simplified?

4. Did the interval stretching portions of the routine help your needs? _____ If so how?

5. Would you be likely to include this type of workout in your exercise program plans?

12.95